50th Anniversary

NME
NEW MUSICAL EXPRESS

CW00336697

Top 100 Singles

The definitive chart of the UK's best-selling songs – EVER

Martin Roach

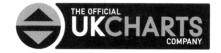

THE OFFICIAL
UKCHARTS
COMPANY

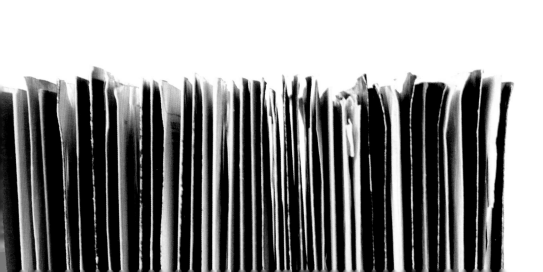

50th Anniversary

NME

NEW MUSICAL EXPRESS

Top 100 Singles

The definitive chart of the UK's best-selling songs – EVER

Martin Roach

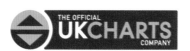

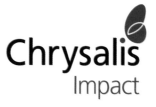

Chrysalis
Impact

First published in 2002 by Chrysalis Impact,
An imprint of Chrysalis Books plc
64, Brewery Road,
London N7 9NT
United Kingdom

© 2002 Chrysalis Books plc
A member of **Chrysalis** Books plc
ISBN 1 84411 006 0

Text © Martin Roach 2002
Volume © Chrysalis Books plc 2002

Credits
Commissioning editors: Will Steeds, Chris Stone
Project management: Laura Ward
Additional research: Darren Haynes
Designed by: Grade Design Consultants, London
Colour reproduction by: Berkeley Square
Printed and bound in: Spain
Singles list compilers: Alan Jones, Tony Brown
Production by: Kerry Tweed

All text and illustrations from NME © IPC Media Limited. Material provided by NME™

Disclaimer
The Top 100 Chart of the UK's Best-Selling Singles was compiled from a combination of sales data provided by The Official UK Charts Company and internal sales information confidentially provided by record companies, together with estimates and algorithms relating to a record's longevity and chart position. While every effort has been made to ensure accuracy, the Publisher and Chart Compilers cannot be held responsible for any errors contained in or omissions from this list, or for any consequences arising therefrom.

The definitive chart of the UK's best-selling songs – EVER...

'Why publish another book of the best singles ever?', I hear you cry. Simple: because *this is the only one that counts*.

This list has been compiled strictly on the basis of the number of singles each entry has sold. Using such a clinical criterion to quantify the fiery and subjective medium of music has thrown up many intriguing and at times perplexing results. You might find that some of the bedfellows are a little odd, but it is a simple fact that, for example, 'Barbie Girl' by Aqua outsold The Beatles' 'Can't Buy Me Love'. Strange, but true.

Researching and writing this book was a mighty challenge indeed – but certainly not an arduous one. Each day brought a new entry and with it fresh anecdotes, even stranger tales of personal success or gritty perseverance, lashings of creative genius or enviable slices of commercial good fortune. As the book was being written, the one hundred songs seemed to come to life in front of me, highlighting some of the highs and lows of the history of rock and roll, the ebb and flow of this most compelling of all art forms.

The final list is a peculiar yet quite brilliant chronicle of the finest, oddest, simplest, most sophisticated and strikingly crafted examples of what music has to offer. I hope you find it as fascinating to read as it was to write.

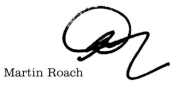

Martin Roach

Contents

The Countdown, the Hit Parade, the Official UK Top 40 – call it what you will, for half a century now, the Official UK Singles Chart has been the backbone of our entertainment culture, part of our everyday language and an important part of our musical heritage.

The first-ever chart – a curious Top 12, listing 15 songs – appeared in the *New Musical Express* on 14 November 1952; Al Martino's 'Here In My Heart' occupied the coveted No. 1 position.

In those days, the chart was compiled by a simple telephone poll of a few record stores. Today, The Official UK Charts Company electronically contacts over 5,000 retail outlets; it is the largest, most sophisticated and accurate piece of weekly market research data in Europe.

Anyone growing up in the UK with even a vague interest in music will have fond memories of the music in the charts. It reflects the era to which we belong – 'date stamping' us – and its tunes travel with us throughout our lives.

Taken together, this phenomenal collection of the Top 100 Best-Selling songs of the past 50 years has clocked up over 2,400 weeks in the Official Top 75 and well over 132 million unit sales.

For the first time ever, The Official UK Charts Company is proud to present this uniquely comprehensive list of the best-sellers, and acknowledges the artists, the record industry and retailers for their contribution in making the Official Singles Chart as exciting and relevant today as it has always been. Here's to the next 50 years.

Omar Maskatiya
Chart Director

Darren Haynes
Brand Marketing Manager

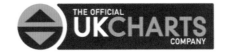

They say the simplest ideas are the best. But when Mr Maurice Kinn and his editorial team came up with the notion of publishing a weekly chart based on singles sales, they surely couldn't have envisaged the amazing institution that the chart would become.

Mr Kinn took over the *New Musical Express* in 1952, legend has it as part payment for a debt he was owed. At that point in time, *NME* was jazz-oriented, served the music industry more than music fans, and was on its uppers. Mr Kinn, quite understandably, was alarmed about this and concocted the mad idea that, if you could find out what music fans were buying, you could write about those records and the stars who were making them. And maybe then more people would buy the paper.

The hunch paid off. *NME* published the first weekly singles chart in the world in November 1952 and the paper's circulation boomed as the writers religiously covered, in turn, Sinatra, Elvis, The Beatles, The Rolling Stones, The Monkees . . . the rest, as you know, is history.

Today the chart is pretty much the same as it's always been – a handy barometer of the most popular songs of the moment. We here at *NME* may not always like what we see when we get the chart on a Sunday, and we may even occasionally pretend to ourselves that it doesn't matter. But it is always a source of jubilation when a song that we like suddenly pops up in the Top Ten and disappointment if it bombs. We, like all music fans, love the thrill of competition that the chart provides.

Here's to another 50 years of classics and duffers and hours of arguments over which is which.

Steve Sutherland
Editorial director, *NME*

50th Anniversary
NME
NEW MUSICAL EXPRESS

The Story of The Charts

The charts are the perennial subject of the 'music's dying' debate – a tired and rather listless argument that seems to fill many column inches each year. This is, of course, utter nonsense. The year 2002 alone has provided two entries which sit very high up on the best-sellers list: Will Young's 'Anything Is Possible/Evergreen' (see No. 12) has achieved sales of 1,779,938, while Gareth Gates' 'Unchained Melody' (see No. 38) has sold 1,318,714 copies to date. So, if new music is keeping the industry vibrant, what

'I don't know what it is. I just fell into it, really. My daddy and I were laughing about it the other day. He looked at me and said, "What happened, El? The last thing I can remember is I was working in a can factory, and you were driving a truck." We all feel the same way about it still. It just . . . caught us up.'
Elvis Presley, 1956

about the role of the charts? Are they less important? In a word, no.

The British have always had a curious yet passionate love affair with the 'hit parade' that shows no signs of cooling off. The popularity of that weekly institution, *Top of the Pops*, is indicative of this enduring fascination with the single. The BBC launched this flagship music programme in January 1964. The first show opened with The Rolling Stones singing 'I Wanna Be Your Man' and was presented by Jimmy Savile. At the time, The Beatles' 'I Want

The very first Top Twelve as published in the *New Musical Express*:

1 **Al Martino** 'Here in My Heart'

2 **Jo Stafford** 'You Belong To Me'

3 **Nat King Cole** 'Somewhere Along The Way'

4 **Bing Crosby** 'Isle Of Innisfree'

5 **Guy Mitchell** 'Feet Up'

6 **Rosemary Clooney** 'Half As Much'

7= **Vera Lynn** 'Forget Me Not'
7= **Frankie Lane** 'High Noon'

8= **Doris Day & Frankie Lane** 'Sugarbush'
8= **Ray Martin** 'Blue Tango'

9 **Vera Lynn** 'Homing Waltz'

10 **Vera Lynn** 'Auf Wiedersehen'

11= **Mario Lanza** 'Because You're Mine'
11= **Max Bygraves** 'Cowpuncher's Cantata'

12 **Johnnie Ray** 'Walking My Baby Back Home'

To Hold Your Hand' was at No. 1 (see No. 14), alongside five other Fab Four hits in the Top 20. To this day, no pop star can persuade his or her curious relatives and disdainful parents that music is 'a proper job' unless he or she has been on 'the Pops'. Why? Because Britain is still infatuated with the pop charts.

The affair started back in 1952 when, on 14 November of that year, *NME* published the first chart. The debut listing was compiled by Percy Dickins, joint founder of *NME*, who personally telephoned a selection of record stores in order to collate his information. The very first No. 1 position was scooped by Al Martino's 'Here In My Heart'. At this stage, only twelve record entries were listed – although this first Top Twelve actually contained fifteen titles, as a number of singles tied for their positions.

Britain back in 1952 was a very different country from the media-savvie, web-surfing, mobile-texting nation that became hypnotised by *Pop Idol* in 2002. In 1952, the accession to the throne of Queen Elizabeth II followed the death in mid-life of the young princess's father, George VI, aged only 57. The world's first nuclear accident at a Canadian atomic research centre threw up a deadly radioactive cloud. In the world of showbusiness, Gene Kelly's legendary performance of the song 'I'm Singin' in the Rain' from the film of the same name marked what many now see as the peak of the musical movie. *The Mousetrap* opened at The Ambassadors Theatre in London's West End for the first of a record-breaking run of shows; the play remains one of the few entertainment 'institutions' that can rival the charts for longevity.

NME POLL — ALL THE WINNERS !

Their pictures are below, and the full results are on page 3

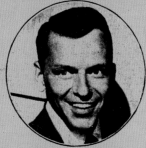

FRANK SINATRA
Outstanding Popular Singer in the World
and Top American Male Singer

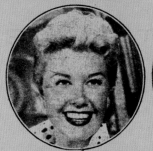

DORIS DAY
Top American Female Singer

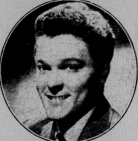

DICKIE VALENTINE
Musical Personality of the Year and
Top Male Solo Singing Star

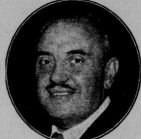

TED HEATH
Top Large Band

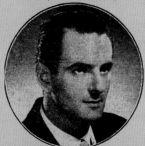

RONNIE SCOTT
Most Promising New Band

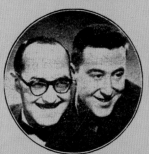

THE KIRCHINS
Top Small Band

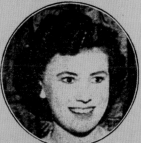

RUBY MURRAY
Top Female Solo Singing Star

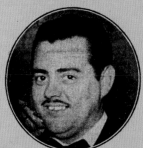

EDDIE CALVERT
Musician of the Year

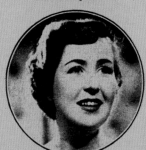

ROSE BRENNAN
Top Female Dance Band Vocalist

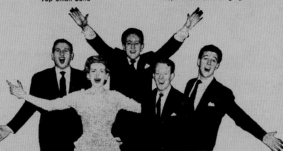

THE STARGAZERS—Top Vocal Group

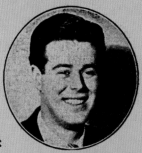

BOBBIE BRITTON
Top Male Dance Band Vocalist

By 1960, the chart was being compiled by *Record Retailer*, later to become *Music Week*. By 1969, sales data from 250 stores was being collated – by hand – to produce the first industry chart. In 2002, chart compilers The Official UK Charts Company use over 5,000 outlets nationwide (representing 99 per cent of the UK's total singles market) and hi-tech computer systems.

Although the *NME* list was initially the sole chart, there are now several other listings available. However, the definitive chart remains the one compiled by The Official UK Charts Company and aired by BBC Radio One on Sunday nights. Other charts use different criteria, such as airplay, to quantify their hits, but the official chart – on which the list in this book is based – is entirely sales driven.

In such a fiery medium as rock 'n' roll, characterised as it is by ever-changing cycles of fashion, it should come as no surprise that the role of the charts has also changed dramatically since its inception. For a time, a new entry at No. 1 was a genuine rarity, which would inevitably attract headlines. Now, such an achievement is almost commonplace. Singles used to chart low and work their way up into the Top Ten. Now, the chart sees an approximate turnover of 50 per cent each week, with most new entries coming in the Top 20.

The figures have changed, too. While we still get the occasional mega-hit – relative newcomers Will Young and Gareth Gates enjoyed startling sales with both of their debut singles – the total number of singles needing to be sold in order to enter the Top 40 has dipped.

There are numerous reasons for these changes. The increasing occurrence of record piracy, CD-burning technology, MP3s, Internet file-swapping and even the cost of singles are just some of the factors quoted by many as contributing to the current fall in singles sales. However, nothing is ever static – the industry has seen declines before, and there is no reason why the current trend should not be reversed.

Some industry observers have tried to dilute the charts' importance still further. In interviews to promote the first single from his 2002 *Heathen* album, David Bowie preferred to call the release a 'radio lead-off track'. Such a view is symptomatic of Bowie's American base, where albums are the defining criteria of success and where singles sales of above ten thousand are unusual. However, this does not signify that the US consumer is unwilling to buy singles *per se*; Stateside, labels took the conscious decision not to release singles, and this move has not been a total success.

In spite of all this, it remains a fact that record companies still look to a Top 40 entry as the criterion by which many acts are classed as successes or failures. This is particularly true with the ultra-expensive pop acts, where a Top 20 – or preferably a Top Ten – slot is needed. In the more alternative world, a Top 40 hit is still seen as a cause for celebration, even if the emphasis *is* on the accompanying album. In defiance of all these doom-mongers, music lovers still walk into a record store and scour the chart lists on the walls to see what to buy. Bands still release singles from albums. MTV still airs thousands of new videos for singles

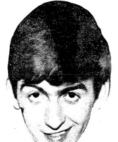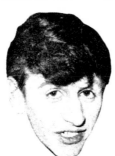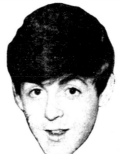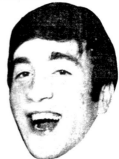
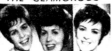
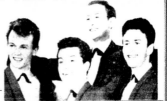
CHELTENHAM, Odeon   Fri. Nov. 1st, 6.30 & 8.45   EXETER, A.B.C.   Thur. Nov. 14th, 6.15 & 8.30   YORK, Rialto   Wed. Nov. 27th, 6.40 & 8.45

15

every year. *Top of the Pops* is still with us. The charts still matter.

Perhaps some of the figures in this list – particularly those in the Top Ten – will never be surpassed. Certainly, Sir Elton John's accomplishment is a unique feat, combining as it does a historically pivotal event with a classic song that seemed magically to assuage the nation's grief. It is unlikely that this staggering achievement – sales nearly 40 per cent greater than the No. 2 record in this list – will ever be matched or beaten, but never say never . . .

This remarkable success is a perfect example of how many of the singles in this list are directly associated with charities, disasters or a 'crunch' moment in history. At times such as these, the British public seems overwhelmed by an inexplicable compulsion to buy a single. Singles are a vital and much-loved part of our cultural heritage and are woven into the very fabric of modern life.

There are numerous other trends highlighted by this list. The correlation between blockbuster films and huge hit singles can reap colossal commercial dividends – here, most successfully with 'You're The One That I Want' (see No. 6) but also, for example, with No.'s 11, 13, 18, 21, 36, 39, 43, 80, 91 and 92. Television also makes its mark (see No.'s 9, 17, 63, 65 and 75). Other songs in this list have received delayed boosts from subsequent inclusion in a film. 'Bohemian Rhapsody' (see No. 3) enjoyed a fresh revival thanks to the Mike Myers comedy smash, *Wayne's World*. Consider also No.'s 40 (*Small Soldiers*), 50 (*Donnie Brasco*) and 57 (*Coneheads*). The weary shoulders of a million pestered parents can be felt by the inclusion of novelty children's hits performed by 'acts' such as Teletubbies and Bob The Builder (see No.'s 60 and 72). Advertising has helped (see No.'s 61 and 81), although the omission of rediscovered classics such as 'I Heard It Through The Grapevine' for the now-renowned Levi's advertisements perhaps puts the power of 'advert exposure' into perspective.

Singles tied to specific events can sell in vast quantities, most obviously, Elton John's 'Candle In The Wind 97' but, in addition, songs such as 'Do They Know It's Christmas?' and 'Perfect Day' (No.'s 2 and 17) have also, somehow, captured the country's collective imagination and tapped into a national conscience to reap such huge sales figures. Where would we be without 'charidee', mate? The Top Ten is fascinating, too: there are no entries from the '50s and only one entry from the '60s. Half of these élite ten singles are from the '70s – the 'daddy' of the big seller.

There are, of course, some surprising omissions from the list: Abba ('Dancing Queen'), The Police ('Every Breath You Take'), or any one of dozens of singles by Madonna, Prince or U2. What about Donna Summer, Bruce Springsteen, The Rolling Stones, The Who, Bob Dylan, Bob Marley, Nirvana, Diana Ross, Tina Turner, The Smiths, REM, Sex Pistols, Mariah Carey, Dire Straits, Jimi Hendrix and Dolly Parton? Of course, many of these names would cry 'We're album artists!' and indeed they are. Nonetheless, their absence is still surprising when Robson Green and Jerome Flynn are flying high in the Top Ten.

Then there are the classic singles which simply did not sell enough to be included in this list: Sinead O' Connor's 'Nothing Compares 2 U', Robbie Williams' 'Angels', 'I Heard It Through The Grapevine' by Marvin Gaye, 'Whiter Shade of Pale' by Procol Harum, 'Bridge Over Troubled Water' by Simon & Garfunkel, 'I Will Survive' by Gloria Gaynor, 'You'll Never Walk Alone' by Gerry and the Pacemakers, 'Hello' by Lionel Richie and, yes, 'Lady In Red' by Chris de Burgh.

Many genres are also notable for their absence – for example, punk, reggae, soul and jungle. However, the veritable 'melting pot' that has been the music scene over the past fifty years means, obviously, that there are inflections of seemingly every style within these one hundred best-selling songs.

For every artist, song and genre I've mentioned above, each reader of this book will be able to find dozens more. That is the beauty of music: it is its subjectivity that keeps the flame alive. This is also why this list was compiled using ONLY sales figures, to ensure absolute parameters in a medium that thrives on the subjective. Such clinical figures highlight the disparity between what is critically revered and what sells record-breaking quantities. Yet, while Tight Fit might not make it into most people's own Rock And Roll Hall of Fame, their contribution and achievement, in terms of appealing to a huge market, should not be underestimated. Therein lies the enduring fascination.

Read it and weep, or read it and remember, whichever is your fancy . . .

NME TOP THIRTY

(Wednesday, November 20, 1963)

Last Week	This		
2	1	SHE LOVES YOU	Beatles (Parlophone)
1	2	YOU'LL NEVER WALK ALONE	Gerry and the Pacemakers (Columbia)
5	3	DON'T TALK TO HIM	Cliff Richard (Columbia)
8	4	I'LL KEEP YOU SATISFIED	Billy J. Kramer (Parlophone)
3	5	SUGAR AND SPICE	Searchers (Pye)
6	6	SECRET LOVE	Kathy Kirby (Decca)
13	7	YOU WERE MADE FOR ME	Freddie and the Dreamers (Columbia)
4	8	BE MY BABY	Ronettes (London)
12	9	MARIA ELENA	Los Indios Tabajaras (RCA)
9	10	BLUE BAYOU	Roy Orbison (London)
7	10	I Shirley Bassey (Columbia)	
10	12	MEMPHIS TENNESSEE	Chuck Berry (Pye Int.)
19	13	IT'S ALMOST TOMORROW	Mark Wynter (Pye)
16	14	BLOWIN' IN THE WIND	Peter, Paul & Mary (Warner Bros.)
14	15	FOOLS RUSH IN	Rick Nelson (Brunswick)
15	16	THEN HE KISSED ME	Crystals (London)
11	17	DO YOU LOVE ME	Brian Poole and the Tremeloes (Decca)
—	17	I ONLY WANT TO BE WITH YOU	Dusty Springfield (Philips)
17	19	IF I HAD A HAMMER	Trini Lopez (Reprise)
—	20	MONEY	Bern Elliott and the Fenmen (Decca)
24	20	YOUR MOMMA'S OUT OF TOWN	Carter-Lewis (Oriole)
—	20	DEEP PURPLE	Nino Tempo and April Stevens (London)
21	23	I WANNA BE YOUR MAN	Rolling Stones (Decca)
27	24	BEATLES VOL. 1 (EP)	Beatles (Parlophone)
28	25	MISS YOU	Jimmy Young (Columbia)
20	26	BUSTED Ray Charles (HMV)	
—	27	GLAD ALL OVER	Dave Clark Five (Columbia)
17	27	THE FIRST TIME	Adam Faith (Parlophone)
—	29	TWIST AND SHOUT (EP)	Beatles (Parlophone)
—	30	BEATLES HITS (EP)	Beatles (Parlophone)

BEST SELLING POP RECORDS IN U.S.

by courtesy of "Billboard"
(Tuesday, November 19, 1963)

Last Week	This		
4	1	I'M LEAVING IT UP TO YOU	Dale & Grace
2	2	WASHINGTON SQUARE	Village Stompers
1	3	DEEP PURPLE	Nino Tempo & April Stevens
7	4	SUGAR SHACK	Jimmy Gilmer & the Fireballs
5	5	IT'S ALL RIGHT	Impressions
3	6	SHE'S A FOOL	Lesley Gore
9	7	EVERYBODY	Tommy Roe
8	8	BOSSA NOVA BABY	Elvis Presley
10	9	DOMINIQUE	Singing Nun
6	10	MARIA ELENA	Los Indios Tabajaras
16	11	PAPA JOE'S	Dixiebelles
15	12	WALKING THE DOG	Rufus Thomas
18	13	HEY LITTLE GIRL	Major Lance
10	14	500 MILES AWAY FROM HOME	Bobby Bare
—	15	LITTLE RED ROOSTER	Sam Cooke
13	16	FOOLS RUSH IN	Rick Nelson
11	17	MEAN WOMAN BLUES	Roy Orbison
—	18	WONDERFUL SUMMER	Robin Ward
—	19	BE TRUE TO YOUR SCHOOL	Beach Boys
—	20	SINCE I FELL FOR YOU	Lenny Welch

BEST SELLING SHEET MUSIC IN BRITAIN

(Tuesday, November 19, 1963)

Last Week	This		
1	1	YOU'LL NEVER WALK ALONE	(Williamson)
3	2	SUGAR AND SPICE	(Welbeck)
2	3	SHE LOVES YOU	(Northern Songs)
5	4	MEMPHIS TENNESSEE	(Jewel)
4	5	MISS YOU	(Campbell-Connelly)
6	6	I	(Shapiro-Bernstein)
10	7	FROM RUSSIA WITH LOVE	(United Artists)
9	8	BLOWIN' IN THE WIND	(Blossom)
17	9	SECRET LOVE	(Harms Witmark)
8	10	DO YOU LOVE ME	(Dominion)
—	11	I'LL KEEP YOU SATISFIED	(Northern Songs)
8	12	IF I HAD A HAMMER	(Essex)
—	12	DON'T TALK TO HIM	(Shadows Music)
11	14	BE MY BABY	(Belinda)
13	15	BLUE BAYOU	(Acuff-Rose)
13	16	STILL	(Peter Maurice)
23	17	YOU WERE MADE FOR ME	(Feldman)
13	18	THE FIRST TIME	(Freddie Poser)
20	19	FOOLS RUSH IN	(Cavendish)
22	20	IF I RULED THE WORLD	(Sterling)
—	21	MONEY	(Dominion)
19	22	HELLO LITTLE GIRL	(Northern Songs)
—	23	MARIA ELENA	(Latin-American)
—	24	IT'S ALMOST TOMORROW	(Macmelodies)
—	25	APPLEJACK	(Essex)
27	25	APPLEJACK	(Essex)
21	26	AIN'T GONNA KISS YA	(Campbell-Connelly)
—	27	WHERE HAVE ALL THE FLOWERS GONE	(Essex)
26	28	EVERYBODY	(Chappell)
—	29	SWEET IMPOSSIBLE YOU	(Peter Maurice)
—	30	TWIST AND SHOUT	(Sherwin)

1 | Candle In The Wind 97/Something About The Way You Look Tonight
Elton John

Release Date: 20.09.97
No. Weeks In Chart: 24
Reached No. 1: 20.09.97
Total Sales: 4,864,611

'I stand before you today the representative of a family in grief, in a country in mourning before a world in shock.'

The opening line from Earl Spencer's funeral address for Diana, Princess of Wales

If one of music's finest attributes is to reflect certain moments in time, then this song is deservedly the biggest-selling single in British (and world) chart history. On 31 August 1997, the UK woke up to the news that Diana, Princess of Wales, the world's most famous woman who'd been hounded by, and yet immersed in, the media, was dead. She was killed by injuries sustained in a high-speed car crash in a central Paris underpass shortly before midnight the day before.

The exact circumstances of the crash generated massive debate about celebrity privacy, the paparazzi and even numerous conspiracy theories. Despite having at times polarised British public opinion, the loss of Diana caused the country to be swept up in scenes of unprecedented national grief.

Elton John was a close personal friend of Diana and, with his lyricist and songwriting partner Bernie Taupin, set about penning a tribute to the mourned Princess. The song they chose to re-work had been composed originally as a tribute to Marilyn Monroe; it only reached No.11 on its first release in 1974. Oddly, the B-side, 'Bennie and the Jets', was released as a

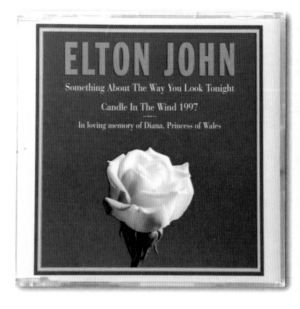

single in America, where it topped the chart. A subsequent live version of 'Candle In The Wind' had reached No. 5 in the UK in 1988.

This 1997 tribute was actually the B-side to Elton's new single, 'Something About The Way You Look Tonight', from his forthcoming album *The Big Picture*. Elton debuted the re-worded

'With just himself at the piano, this was possibly the most highly pressured live performance in history.'

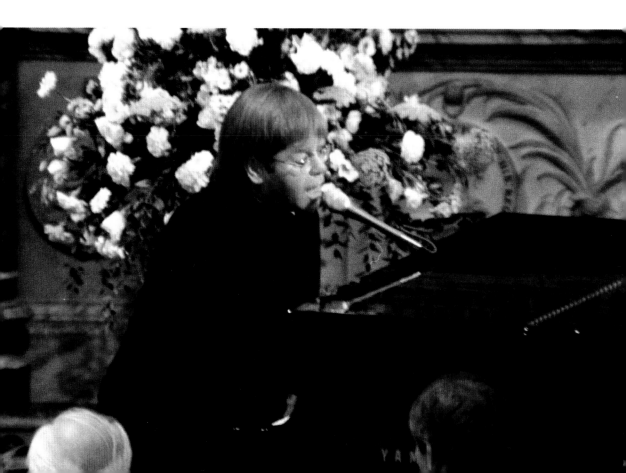

version at the funeral of Diana – with just himself at the piano, this was possibly the most highly pressured live performance in history. Equal credit must go to John's lyricist, Bernie Taupin, whose poetic new words belied the slim time frame allowed for him to re-sculpt an acknowledged classic.

The public, massed in their thousands outside Westminster Abbey and watching in their millions at home, listened to the references to 'England's rose' and the 'greenest hills' as Elton both expressed their shared grief and also offered the country a metaphorical shoulder to cry on. Within minutes of the rendition, the public was demanding that the song become commercially available.

This version of the song was produced by Beatles cohort Sir George Martin in just one day and then rush-released for mid-September, 1997, only two weeks after Diana's death. Even allowing for the circumstances in which it was released, few could have guessed at the exact scale of the forthcoming phenomenon. The statistics are unparalleled, even by sales giants such as Band Aid and 'Bohemian Rhapsody' (see No.'s 2, 3). The single was released on a Saturday, so without the luxury of a full week's sales, but still entered at No. 1 after selling 658,000 copies in one day. (George Michael's 'You Have Been Loved/The Sweetest Thing' charted at No. 2 but was outsold by seven to one.) Apart from Band Aid's first-week tally of 750,000 copies, this single-day total exceeded that of any other song sold in seven days. The vast majority of the single's UK total of 4.86 million came within five weeks of its release.

Also in this year . . .

* Puff Daddy's tribute to his friend Notorious B.I.G, splicing a sample of The Police's 'Every Breath You Take', was a worldwide No. 1 smash.
* The Spice Girls exported Girl Power en masse and achieved the unthinkable by cracking America.
* Essex hard dance act The Prodigy became only the seventh British group to enter the US album charts at No. 1 thanks to their ten-million-selling *Fat of the Land*.
* Kylie Minogue enjoyed a brief mini-revival with two Top 30 singles, but most observers felt that her career was in permanent decline.
* A re-issue of Elvis Presley's 'Always On My Mind' re-entered the charts, going straight in at No. 13.

The song also became the US's fastest-selling single ever, with first-week figures of 3.4 million units (from advance orders of eight million, on its way to eleven million). This was a remarkable five times the 632,000 of previous record holder Whitney Houston's 'I Will Always Love You'. The record was No. 1 in almost every country where charts were compiled – in Canada, it was in the Top 20 for three years, with 45 weeks at the top. Obviously Elton's biggest hit, a grand total of 33 million sales raised £20 million for the Diana, Princess of

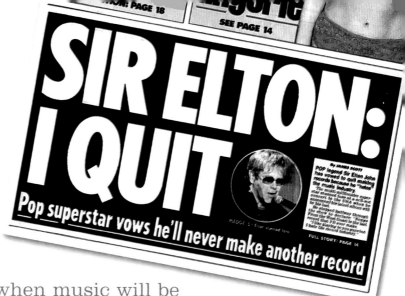

'The threat of a year when music will be dominated by a sense of mass guilt, when consensus rock will patronise and prey on traditional British gullibility, plainly impinges on our world.'

John Mulvey, *NME,* **20 September 1997.**

Wales, Memorial Fund. Yet, despite all this commercial success, 1997 was in many ways an awful year for Elton, who had already grieved for his murdered friend, Italian fashion designer Gianni Versace.

Elton had first met Bernie Taupin when they both answered a 1967 record company advertisement in *New Musical Express*. Alongside battles with drug addiction and other personal problems, Elton went on to create a revered canon of work in the early '70s, which included seminal songs such as 'Rocket Man',

'Daniel', 'Goodbye Yellow Brick Road' and the original rendition of 'Candle In The Wind'. With a vast personal fortune and 40 hit albums behind him, Elton is a genuine musical legend. He remains the only UK artist to debut at No.1 in the US singles chart, and can boast more record sales than any other British solo male performer. It is unlikely that this single will ever be replaced as the world's biggest seller. In early 1998, Elton John was knighted, during which ceremony at Buckingham Palace he was mistakenly announced as 'Sir John Elton'.

2

Do They Know It's Christmas?
Band Aid

Release Date: 15.12.84
No. Weeks In Chart: 20
Reached No. 1: 15.12.84
Total Sales: 3,550,000

Geldof almost single-handedly organised every aspect of the recording, from 'phoning superstars to booking studio time and arranging engineers.

Former journalist and lead singer with Irish band The Boomtown Rats, Bob Geldof was sitting in his London flat watching a BBC report on African famine, narrated by Michael Buerke and filmed by Mohamed Amin. Faced with such an appalling spectre of near-biblical proportions, Geldof was deeply disturbed and promptly flew out to Ethiopia to inspect the suffering for himself. Horrified by what he saw, he came back to England and, with long-time friend and fellow pop star/songwriter, Midge Ure of Ultravox, penned this historically significant song.

Geldof was famous for his very direct personality; but the passion with which he corralled over 40 of the UK's biggest pop stars into SARM Studios, West London, to record this single, swept the whole nation up in a tidal wave of excitement.

The Sunday morning of 25 November 1984 saw a recording session with no celebrity tantrums, no late arrivals and no egotistical demands – all present had to take any complaints to an impassioned Geldof. No one

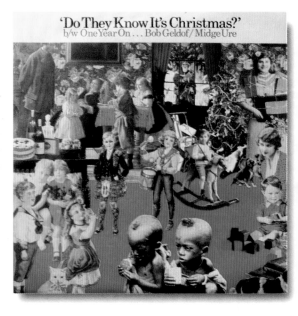

'Do They Know It's Christmas?'
b/w One Year On . . . Bob Geldof / Midge Ure

did. Rumour has it that when America's own charity single, 'We Are The World', was stumbling amid personality clashes, schedule problems and other issues, Geldof went in, SAS-style, to blast the problems out (the UK song

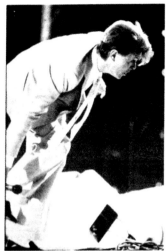

Bowie stoops to conquer.

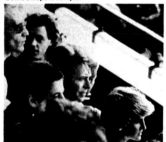

Bob, Dave and Di: Saint, Duke and Princess.

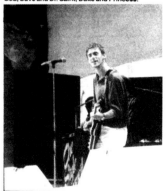

Internationalist goes worldwide.

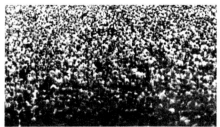

The Hallowed Turf from the Royal Box.

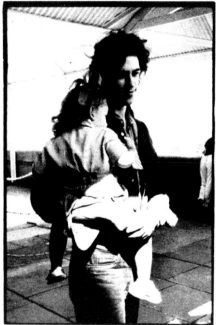

A moment of peace.

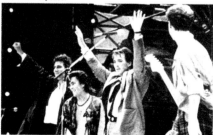

Spandau: up and away.

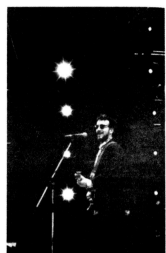

Old Northern English folk singer.

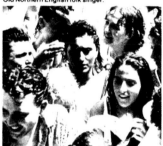

2.15, the heat is on.

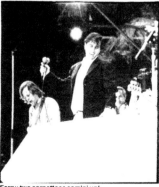

Ferry: two cornettoes comin' up!

was also a major hit in the US, albeit not until the following January).

Although the song was only No. 1 for five weeks, the vast quantities being sold each day very quickly racked up much of its staggering total. Such sales kept the impressive popularity of Wham!'s single, 'Last Christmas', off the No. 1 slot – George Michael later donated his band's royalties from that single to Geldof's project.

The record had been launched with a concert at the Royal Albert Hall, but Geldof's plans were already on a much grander scale. His thoughts had turned to staging a gigantic concert, to be called Live Aid. So he compiled the greatest billing ever witnessed – only Prince (retired from public performance), Bruce Springsteen (reluctantly unavailable due to severe touring commitments) and Michael Jackson (reason unknown) were absent. The Who and Led Zeppelin reformed, as did Black Sabbath.

Wembley Stadium was complemented by a parallel show in Philadelphia. It was watched by 1.5 billion people and raised another £70 million, the largest charity sum collected by one single event. Much of the reason for the financial success stemmed from Bob's demand that everyone involved supply their services for free (as they had with the single). British Telecom offered twenty free phone lines; Geldof wanted a thousand. He won.

In the aftermath of the greatest concert the world is ever likely to see (the end of which saw an embarrassed but intensely proud Geldof hoisted on the shoulders of Paul McCartney and Pete Townshend), this single went back to the No. 3 slot. It is an annual Christmas seller,

resulting in accumulative sales of a staggering 3.55 million. The PWL-produced Band Aid 2, featuring Bros, Kylie Minogue, Rick Astley, Jason Donovan and Bananarama among others, reached No.1 in 1989 (with the original version as a B-side).

Geldof was nominated for the Nobel Peace Prize and in 1986 he was also rewarded with a knighthood. His initial aim had been to raise £72,000 from this single – it generated £8 million. The Band Aid foundation, when it closed down in 1992, had collected over £100 million. Only two per cent went on administration, the remainder went on either immediate or long-term aid.

Also in this year . . .

* Status Quo finally 'split up' after no fewer than 22 years on the road.
* Marvin Gaye was shot dead by his retired father the day before his 45th birthday.
* Alison Moyet and Sade vied with each other as the nation's most popular female soloists.
* Maverick performer Cyndi Lauper enjoyed her debut hit with 'Girls Just Want To Have Fun'.
* Germany's hirsute-armpitted Nena topped the charts with her rock pop classic, '99 Red Balloons'.

HARVEY GOLDSMITH, BOB GELDOF AND MAURICE JONES FOR THE BAND AID TRUST PRESENT

AT
WEMBLEY STADIUM
LONDON

ADAM ANT
BOOMTOWN RATS
DAVID BOWIE
PHIL COLLINS
ELVIS COSTELLO
DIRE STRAITS
BRYAN FERRY
ELTON JOHN
HOWARD JONES
NIK KERSHAW
ALISON MOYET
QUEEN
SADE
SPANDAU BALLET
STATUS QUO
STYLE COUNCIL
STING
U2
ULTRAVOX
PAUL YOUNG
WHAM!
THE WHO

AT
J.F.K. STADIUM
PHILADELPHIA

BRYAN ADAMS
THE CARS
ERIC CLAPTON
DURAN DURAN
BOY GEORGE
HALL AND OATES
MICK JAGGER
BILLY JOEL
WAYLON JENNINGS
JUDAS PRIEST
KRIS KRISTOFFERSON
HUEY LEWIS & THE NEWS
ROBERT PLANT
POWER STATION
PRETENDERS
SANTANA
PAUL SIMON
SIMPLE MINDS
TEARS FOR FEARS
TEMPTATIONS
THOMPSON TWINS
NEIL YOUNG
STEVIE WONDER

LIVE AID

JULY 13th

DOORS OPEN 10 AM, CONCERT STARTS 12 NOON FINISHES 10 PM
Tickets at £25 are on sale **NOW** from Wembley Stadium Box Office.

And subject to 50p booking fee per ticket at counter sales from
Keith Prowse, Premier London Theatre Bookings, Stargreen Agencies.
And BRIGHTON Centre, GUILDFORD, CROYDON, Fairfront, PORTSMOUTH Guildhall, OXFORD Apollo.
And subject to £1 booking fee per ticket from
Keith Prowse Credit Card No 01-741 8999

SOLD OUT

Or see local press for inclusive coach and concert tickets. Tickets are limited to 6 per person.
DO NOT PAY MORE THAN THE LISTED PRICE FOR YOUR TICKETS.
OUR THANKS TO N.M.E. FOR DONATING THIS PAGE.
NO BOTTLES, NO CANS WILL BE ALLOWED IN THE STADIUM.
**ANY DONATIONS WILL BE GRATEFULLY RECEIVED TO 'BAND AID TRUST'
c/o STOY HAYWARD 8 BAKER STREET, LONDON WIM IDJ.**

3

Bohemian Rhapsody
Queen

Release Date: 8.11.75
No. Weeks In Chart: 31
Reached No. 1: 29.11.75
Total Sales: 2,130,000

> This is Queen's signature song – the most critically revered single ever also enjoys the rare duality of mammoth commercial success.

This song captured the very essence of Queen: their pomposity, their overt campness, their technical brilliance, their brazen ambition and unique genius.

Previous to this landmark record, Queen had enjoyed solid success, but this single, their fourth UK hit, was their first No.1 and the song that would set them on the path to iconic status. Hints of more complex studio work had seeped out on 1974's *Queen 2* but no one expected this, a cod-operatic masterpiece, told in four movements, and using every studio and mixing-desk trick in the book.

The first signs of Freddie's ambitions for the track came when he was explaining the song, which Brian May called 'Freddie's baby', in his flat, and said, 'Now dears, this is where the opera section comes in'. (He revealed later that he had researched opera before starting work on this song.) Recording this vision was, predictably, exhausting, taking three full weeks. The operatic backing vocals alone took Freddie, Brian May and Roger Taylor 70 working hours. Rock legend recalls how the 180 overdubs wore the tapes so thin that at points they were almost transparent. Yet, reportedly, the band was in continual fits of laughter in the studio at the burgeoning campness of the song. The striking changes in tempo were distinctly unorthodox, but somehow dovetailed seamlessly.

This set the tone for the resulting album, *A Night At The Opera*. Queen had set out to record what they called a 'classic' album using state-of-the-art technology, but no synthesisers (their records at this point boasted of a lack of such). They used six studios over five months, making it the most expensive album ever recorded at that point.

Aside from the magnificent musical bombast, vocally the record was a ludicrous slice of genius, especially considering that Freddie had been forced to cancel several shows earlier in the year due to severe throat problems. The

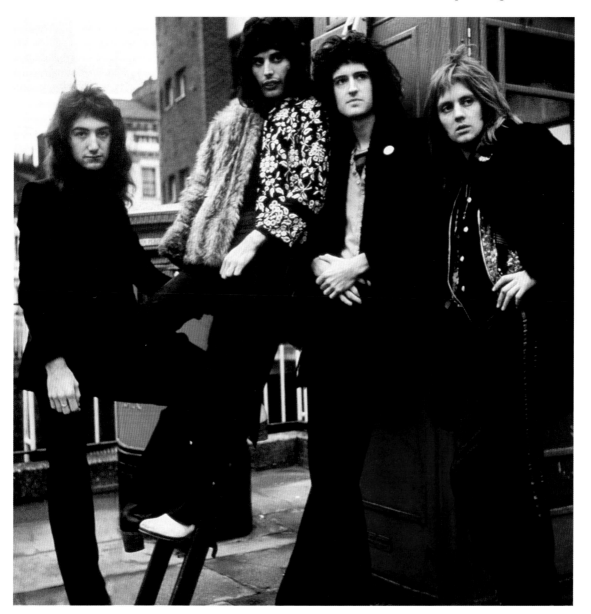

song lurches from raging pathos to deluded defiance and pitiful despair, yet Freddie never revealed his inspiration for the intensely scrutinised lyrics, obtusely saying that they were just 'about relationships'. Without Freddie, the song would have been impossible.

The specially commissioned promotional footage, seen by many as the birth of the modern video, cost just £5,000 and was directed by Bruce Gowers around a concept of the band's own devising. Initially, the Vaudevillian six-minute epic was considered too long for a commercial single release, but the band refused to edit it down. Freddie then gave an acetate copy to his close friend and DJ, Kenny Everett, with strict instructions not to play it on air – which Everett did fourteen times over the next two days (he said his 'finger slipped').

The subsequent public demand was so great that EMI had no choice but to release the single, which was at No. 1 within weeks. In America, the song and album were equally successful, marking Queen out as one of the world's biggest acts. It was perhaps ironic that as punk broke, eschewing as it did the excess of bloated rock, Queen actually delivered the very song that made all the guitar-wielding extravagance make sense.

The statistical achievements of the song are breathtaking. It was No. 1 for nine weeks, selling in excess of one million copies. After Freddie Mercury's death from Aids-related illness in November 1991, a fund-raising release of the original returned to the top spot, again over Christmas (for five weeks), and again selling over a million. Due to the Yuletide timing, it is the only song to be No. 1 in four separate years, accumulating a total of fourteen weeks. In 1992, it gained further popularity when it featured in the classic 'headbanging sketch' in the Mike Myers blockbuster comedy film, *Wayne's World*. More exposure came in the Queen musical, *We Will Rock You*, which opened in 2001. Elton John, Rolf Harris and Weird Al Yankovic are just a few of the artists who have covered this song.

Arguably, no other group could have conceived or executed such a theatrical extravaganza. Thank God that they did.

Also in this year . . .

* Lou Reed had three albums on release: *Rock And Roll Animal II*, *Metal Machine Music* and *Coney Island Baby*.
* John Lennon successfully won access to his own US Department of Immigration file with regard to his forthcoming deportation case.
* Despite a promise to perform in the UK within the next twelve months, Elvis never did – instead, checking into a hospital halfway through a Las Vegas residency.
* Bruce Springsteen broke into the mainstream, admitting he was worried by all the hype surrounding him.
* Pink Floyd played in front of 70,000 people at Knebworth at their own festival, with flypasts by two Spitfires.

QUEEN: Bohemian Rhapsody (EMI). And talking of 10CC, this owes more than a couple of bob to Strawberry Studios — especially in its use of the split cascading chorus, and the elongation of the ends of certain words. The song has four movements of seemingly quite different nature, so it'll be interesting to see whether it'll be played in its entirety on the radio. It's performed extremely well, but more in terms of production than anything else. Charles' point about Springsteen's "Born To Run" also applies here — that someone somewhere has decided that the boys' next release must sound 'epic'. And it does. They sound extremely self-important.

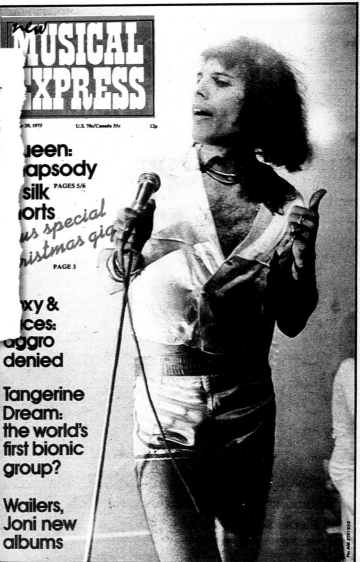

new

MUSICAL EXPRESS

...er 29, 1975   U.S. 70c/Canada 35c   12p

...ueen:
...apsody
...silk   PAGES 5/6
...orts
...us special
...ristmas gig
PAGE 3

...xy &
...ces:
...aggro
denied

Tangerine
Dream:
the world's
first bionic
group?

Wailers,
Joni new
albums

4

Mull of Kintyre/Girls' School
Wings

Release Date: 19.11.77
No. Weeks In Chart: 17
Reached No. 1: 3.12.77
Total Sales: 2,050,000

One of four singles to sell more than two million copies, 'Mull' was co-written by Laine, who later sold his rights to the song to McCartney after being declared bankrupt.

In many ways, 1977 was a muted year, not least because of the death of the two most successful male artists ever – Bing Crosby and Elvis Presley. It was a year full of disco and angry punk, making this song an unlikely smash hit. Recorded at Abbey Road Studios in London, this was a plain eulogy to Paul and Linda McCartney's home or, more specifically, the southern tip of the Kintyre island, some eleven miles from their Campbeltown farm.

A straightforward if not simplistic song, the track defied the critics' disdain to become the then best-selling single in British chart history (only later would further sales of Queen's 1975 classic 'Bohemian Rhapsody' surpass these figures; see No. 3). Set against a backdrop of bagpipes and choral vocals, the song encapsulated the strange dichotomy of life after The Beatles for Paul McCartney. While George Harrison and John Lennon enjoyed some degree of critical acclaim – most notably on the former's *All Things Must Pass* and the latter's *Imagine* – McCartney's post-Fab Four records

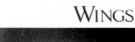

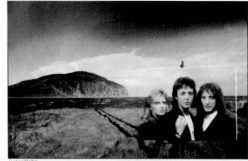

were often universally pilloried. Nonetheless, this single managed to outsell any release by McCartney's three former band mates, and even outperformed The Beatles' best-selling single and previous record holder, 'She Loves You' (see No. 8), by over 16,000 copies.

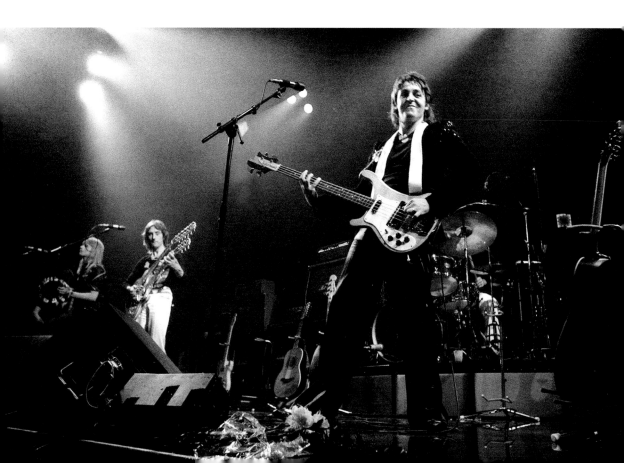

After his engagement with Jane Asher had been broken off, McCartney met and fell in love with American Linda Eastman. The official end of The Beatles had come in April 1970, but by then McCartney was already married to Linda, who would become his very public soul mate over the ensuing years. Their intensely close relationship was one of rock's rare beacon's of fidelity, until her untimely death from breast cancer in 1999. Wings was formed after an initially successful solo album by McCartney and a collaborative one with Linda. Over the years the line-up changed often, but the key members were Paul and Linda, alongside former Moody Blue, Denny Laine.

The early days of Wings saw some strong live shows, including a spate of 'spontaneous' gigs at universities. The first of these, at Nottingham, saw Paul and the band turn up unannounced at the Students' Union with an offer to play that night – this particular concert, in front of 700 stunned students, was his first live show in five years.

By contrast, the critics were quick to pounce on the softer musicality of McCartney's new recorded work. The band's debut album, *Wings Wild Life*, was panned. Wings' greatest acclaim came with 1974's *Band On The Run* long player, which was No. 1 on both sides of the Atlantic. 'Live And Let Die', the theme tune to the James Bond movie of the same name, also enjoyed its share of critical applause.

Nonetheless, the spectre of the now-fabled Lennon/McCartney writing partnership will perhaps always haunt McCartney's post-1970 work. By way of justification, merciless critics cited post-Beatles songs about Paul's jeep and Labrador dog, records such as 'Mary Had A Little Lamb' and his cover of the theme tune to the TV soap opera, *Crossroads*.

'Mull' replaced Abba's 'Name of the Game' at the top and remains unchallenged as 1977's best-seller and the year's only entry in this book. Its nine weeks at No. 1 over the Christmas period was ended, rather oddly, by 'Uptown Top Ranking', the patois-inflected novelty one-hit wonder of Jamaican school girls Althia And Donna. This huge hit was Wings' only No. 1 (with McCartney, surprisingly, only enjoying one genuine solo No. 1 with 1983's 'Pipes of Peace').

The millions of Beatles' disciples in America did not take to the bagpipes, and instead made the more rocking sound of 'Girls' School' the US A-side, but even then the single only reached No. 33 on that side of the Atlantic.

In 1980, McCartney served a ten-day jail sentence in Japan for possession of marijuana, resulting in a Wings tour being cancelled; a set back from which the band never really recovered. In the spring of 1981, Paul announced that the band was no more, shortly after commencing work with Beatles' producer George Martin on 'The Frog Song'.

McCartney was knighted in 1997 and remains the only artist to have enjoyed No. 1 hits as a soloist, in a duet, trio, quartet and quintet. By a strange coincidence, this is the same 'Mull' as that where a Chinook helicopter crashed in 1994, killing 29 senior military personnel and becoming the subject of a protracted government investigation.

Mull of Kintyre is number one.

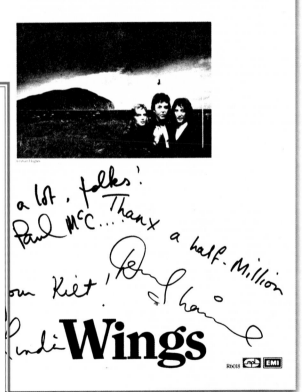

Also in this year . . .

* Elvis Presley died in the bathroom of his Gracelands home on 16 August, moving President Jimmy Carter to pronounce, 'Elvis's death deprives our country of a part of itself.'
* Ozzy Osbourne quit metal forefathers Black Sabbath.
* Peter Gabriel played in his first solo shows since leaving Genesis some two years earlier.
* Virgin Records signed The Sex Pistols in the band's third record deal in under six months.
* Fleetwood Mac released what is widely regarded as the pinnacle of their careers with the album, *Rumours*.

Wings

R6018

5

Rivers Of Babylon/ Brown Girl In The Ring
Boney M

Release Date: 29.04.78
No. Weeks In Chart: 40
Reached No. 1: 13.05.78
Total Sales: 1,985,000

The band's rise to fame in the UK was stalled at first, after the cover for their second album drew criticism for featuring the girls naked and Bobby in his underwear.

Boney M are the only group to hold two of the ten biggest-selling singles in British chart history (see also No. 10). The brainchild of German producer Frank Farian, the band, based in Offenbach, West Germany, was initially a studio creation for filtering session-musician dance tunes into the European underground scene. The group's first official effort was the oddly entitled song 'Baby Do You Wanna Bump?' in 1975, which proved to be an underground hit in Holland and Belgium only.

Following this flicker of success, Farian dropped his early pseudonym Zambi and recruited West Indian Bobby Farrell, Jamaicans Marcia Barrett and Liz Mitchell and Montserrat-born Maizie Williams. Liz Mitchell had moved to Germany in the late '60s and sang in the German version of the musical *Hair*; for many her distinctive voice became synonymous with the band's sound. Taking part of their name from an Australian TV hero, the band began to perform on the German nightclub scene. Within a few months, their debut album, *Take The Heat Off Me*, was that country's best-seller.

The first signs of the looming sales behemoth came when Dutch television shows started to request appearances by Boney M, which in turn generated more club shows. A German TV rendition of 'Daddy Cool' helped Boney M crash into the UK charts at No. 6. This debut hit started an impressive run of nine consecutive Top Ten singles, including the tenth- and fifth-biggest UK sellers ever. A cover of Paul Simon's 'Sunny' followed, launching them into the Top Five and opening the gold lamé floodgates.

As 1978 rolled around, Boney M were about to become massive. A string of Top Ten hits followed before this song became their first No. 1 and career best. Initially released as just 'Rivers of Babylon', a version of the Melodians' original, the song spent so much time in the charts (40 weeks in total, of which five were at

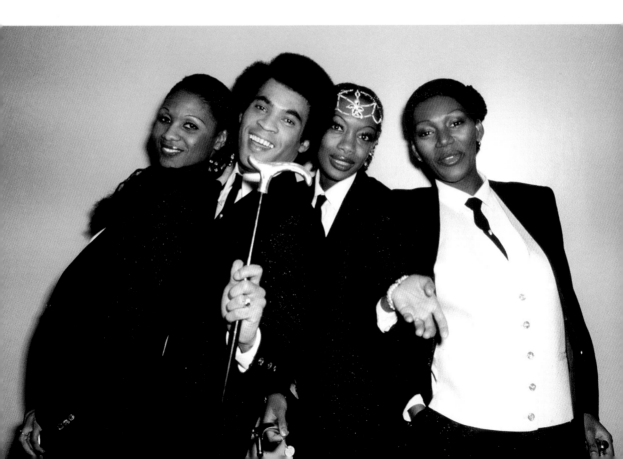

No. 1) that radio stations got bored of playing it and flipped the disc over to air 'Brown Girl In The Ring' instead – a light-hearted disco version of a Jamaican folk song first made famous by Exuma. The single had slid out of the Top 20 but, as soon as radio aired the B-side, it shot back up to No. 1. Despite almost total domination of the UK and European charts (see No. 10), Boney M only saw this one record pierce the US's Top Ten, despite that country's thirst for all things disco.

Demand for this single was so great that eight designated pressing plants could not cope with the surge of orders, and retailers were obliged to resort to shipping in European imports. The 1978 album *Nightflight to Venus* also hit the top (one of three that did so), staying in the charts for 65 weeks. Elsewhere, seven of their songs achieved a No. 1 position across Europe and, by the end of 1978, Farian's few hundred copies of his debut disc had been swelled to over 50 million records.

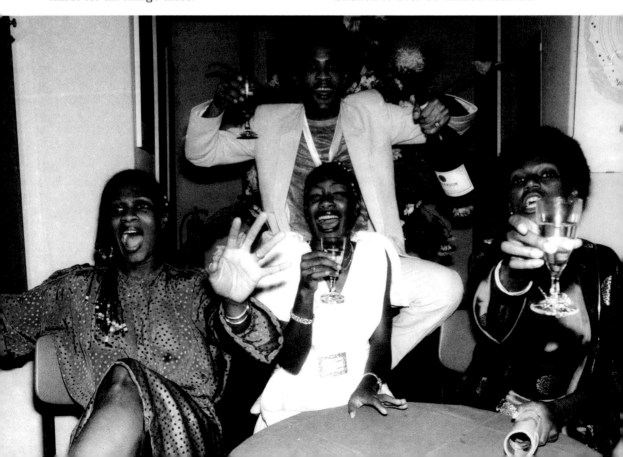

BY THE RIVERS (well...sands, beaches, coves, quays and bays)
OF BABBACOMBE

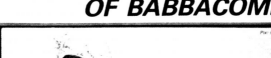

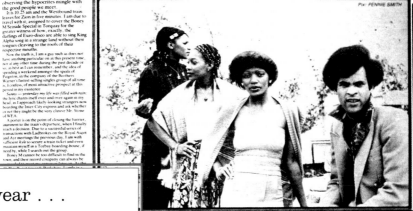

Pix: PENNIE SMITH

...d a thousand disco riffs: L to r, Marcia, Maizie, Liz, Bobby.

Sunny Seaside Special with BONEY M
PENNY REEL sends a postcard

TORBAY OR NOT Torbay — that is the question! I am standing at the barrier of Platform 2, Paddington, one chilly Saturday morning expressing Brandoesque mutterance of this sentiment whilst scoring the station for one whom answers to the description of a WEA liaison officer named Don Stone and/or a quartet of high-stepping black pop stars, three women and one man, called Boney M; observing the hypocrites mingle with the good people we meet.

It is 10.25 am and the Westbound train leaves for Zion in five minutes. I am due to travel with it, assigned to cover the Boney M Seaside Special in Torquay for the greater witness of how, exactly, the darlings of Euro-disco are able to sing King Alpha song in a strange land without their tongues cleaving to the roofs of their respective mouths.

Now the truth is, I am a guy such as does not have anything particular on at this present time, not at any other time during the past decade or so, as best as I can remember, and the idea of spending a weekend amongst the spoils of Paignton, in the company of the Brothers Warner's fastest-selling singles group of all time is, I confess, of most attractive prospect at this period in my existence.

Suns — yesterday my life was filled with rain, the lyric chants itself over and over again in my head, as I approach likely looking strangers now boarding the Inter-City express and ask whether or not they might be the very elusive Mr. Stone of WEA.

A porter is on the point of closing the barrier, moment to the train's departure, when I finally reach a decision. Due to a successful series of transactions with Ladbrokes on the Royal Ascot and Ayr meetings the previous day, I am with sufficient kyle to secure a train ticket and even maintain myself in a Torbay boarding-house, if need by, while I search out the group.

Boney M cannot be too difficult to find in the town, and their record company can always be...

[text continues, partially illegible]

...looks at Don. "This ...ardee man, you know," ...a knot up the dread. Nab ...roots," finishing with a ...anna's hit.

...e. "I hope you're going to ...ich other with a level ...iz explodes into a fit of

...decide I have fallen in love ...o let it happen and enjoy

...Mitchell, born Clarendon, ...Cancer in 1952 is both ...member and also its ...ccessive NME chart hits: ...ny", "Ma Baker", ...Of Babylon", as well as ...heir two Atlantic albums, ...Me" and "Love For Sale". ...berlain Road school in ...been living with her ...s and two sisters in ...ting the German ...ter to having been chosen ...r Frank Farian to lead his

...Rampa as her favourite ...Marvin Gaye and Candi ...ingers; "No Woman No ...bylon", "Daddy's Home" ...Equal Rights" as her ...West Indian her favourite ...New Testament Church of ...o points to the Ras ...ing a petitive — her

Abbey Meadows on the Torquay seafront, where a huge marquee tent announces the presence of a BBC Seaside Special.

The enclosure is thronged with various dancers from Geoff Richer's First Edition, assorted Smokies, Showaddywaddys, friends of Sacha Distel and other Blockheads, including Cosmo Vinyl and Ian Dury — described as a "punk" by Bobby Farrell — and make our way to the Boney M trailer, where we are summarily joined by ravishing, red-headed Austro-Hungarian aristocrat Penny Maclean, lead siren with Boney M's main rival Deutsch disco outfit, Silver Convention.

There follows much hanging about between acts, and fairly soon the small trailer is becoming a wee heady with the spice of preening, perfumed femininity, such as this man's sensibilities finds especially seductive, but since the ensuing conversation never resolves itself upon matters sexual, I grow slightly bored and wander out and into the adjoining marquee where yet a further clot of black, Jamaican disco-chanteuseuses, Black Gold, are discussing the finer details of their stage entrance and general dance routine with the BBC producer for tonight's filming of their TV debut.

Meanwhile, Monsieur Distel is flashing sundry charm to his own inimitable manner, in front of such friends, camera technicians and idle onlookers as may be present, and for their benefit.

Ian Dury and The Blockheads are next. They appear in full stage dress, sporting red, gold and green clothes pegs, bequeathed by Mariambo during the two groups' recent tour of the UK together, and run through a couple of takes of "What A Waste", eagerly attended by an audience of First Edition dancers taking a tea break.

Boney M need little instruction as the group pace the length of a "Daddy Cool"/"Sunny"/"Belfast" medley, followed by a

full-length rendition of "Ma Baker", and in less than a quarter of an hour our quartet are finished for the afternoon, with the ladies collecting their fur wraps from clothes hanger Don Stone.

WE MAKE OUR way back to the New Grand for tea, scones, cheese and the best suave clotted cream any of us have ever tasted. Maizie pulls her fox from her shoulders and declares:

"Bwoy, but it nice to be back in England with all their quaint customs. Really," she puts "high tea in the afternoon. Simply purrfect".

We all fall about giggling at this typical Ms Williams commentary. Liz, taking hold of my hand, remarks through a mouthful of jam and pastry: "Did you ever nyam such beautiful food, Rasta? Hey, man, it's great to be home." She starts to stroke my leg and I begin to dissolve into the clotted cream.

Don Stone asks if we should make plans to arrange a taped interview between the group and myself, but I demur at the prospect of introducing cassette recorders into our cosy little tea party and insist there will be material sufficient for a feature without. A good and serious thing, because right now Marcia is understudying the dormouse in Alice and gradually falling asleep on her consort Eric's shoulder.

"The brother cool," chimes in the normally silent Carl. "He jus' groove in with the vibe." Don man, and him easy. That's the same way I would write an article.

And having thus pronounced this, for Carl abnormally lengthy speech, he disengaged himself from our company and made his passage towards the television room to watch Brazil play Italy in the World Cup. The rest of the company

● Continues page 9

Also in this year . . .

* Disco fever gripped the world.
* The Sex Pistols split up after the debacle of an ill-fated US tour. Sid Vicious was later charged with murdering girlfriend Nancy Spungen.
* The reclusive genius Kate Bush wowed music lovers with her enigmatic debut single, 'Wuthering Heights'.
* Bob Dylan toured the UK for the first time in almost a decade.
* Grateful Dead played three gigs at the Egyptian pyramids of Giza, in front of a nightly audience of 3,000.

...Don introduces us as we depart from the lift ...together. "This is Penny Reel," he explains, ...the journalist who's come to cover the Seaside ...Special for New Musical Express."

"Oh." You the guy we are supposed to meet

OUR NINE-STRONG party leaves the hotel and, to the accompanying stares and Three Degrees conjecture of passing holidaymakers, cross The King's Drive to Torre

You're The One That I Want
John Travolta and
Olivia Newton-John

Release Date: 20.05.78
No. Weeks In Chart: 35
Reached No. 1: 17.06.78
Total Sales: 1,975,000

An antidote to the crumbling punk scene, Newton-John and Travolta's squeaky-clean duet was the biggest-selling of the four singles from the *Grease* soundtrack, and the resounding climax to that hit film.

The year 1978 saw the greatest number of singles sold to date in chart history. Not surprising, perhaps, with the likes of Abba, Boney M, Village People, Kate Bush and other legends all releasing records. The biggest seller of all? John Travolta. Why? *Grease.*

Producer Allan Carr had bought the rights to the Broadway musical *Grease*, initially with Elvis Presley in mind. He then approached the star of the American hit TV show *Happy Days*, Henry Winkler, a.k.a. The Fonz, but 'Fonzy' declined. Frustrated, Carr sat flicking through the channels on his TV when a young, swaggering, cocky 'punk' came onto his screen. It was John Travolta, playing the hugely popular Vinnie Barberino in the ABC comedy series *Welcome Back, Kotter*.

With several TV roles under his belt, the young Travolta had already appeared in theatre, including, ironically, a minor role in the touring company's version of *Grease*. Travolta, the youngest of six children, all in entertainment, was getting 8,000 fan mail letters a week as Barberino and even released his own Top Ten US hit, 'Let Her In', in mid-1976. Blown away by Travolta's screen presence, Carr offered him the lead role of '50s greaser Danny Zuko.

In what must be the most successful stop-gap measure of all-time, Carr placed Travolta in another film he was releasing while production on *Grease* was resolved. The movie, *Saturday Night Fever*, was set against the backdrop of the New York City disco nightlife. It was a global sensation – over 30 million album soundtrack sales and a seismic cultural impact turned Travolta into a superstar.

Travolta's co-star in *Grease* was already something of a superstar. Australian-based Olivia Newton-John, granddaughter of Nobel prize-winning physicist Max Born, was a Grammy-winning country star (on the back of 1973's US No. 1, 'Let Me Be There', written by late Shadow, John Rostill).

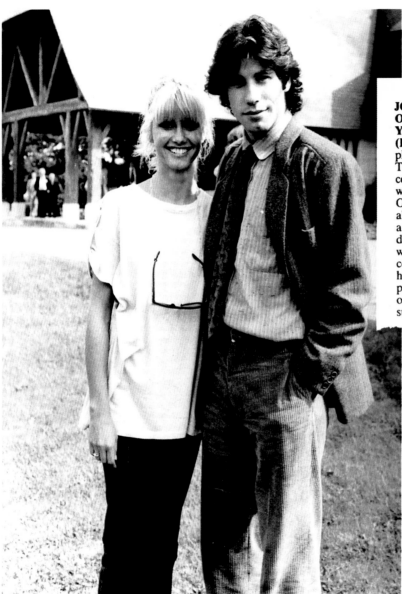

**JOHN TRAVOLTA &
OLIVIA NEWTON-JOHN:
You're The One That I want
(RSO).** From the film of the
play of *Grease,* this proves that
Travolta's singing is about as
convincing as his acting. (He
wiggles his bum nicely, mind).
Olivia is as wonderful as she
always was, and quite probably
a deal richer. I very much
doubt whether 50s rock'n'roll
was anything like this, but
concern for trivialities like
historical authenticity won't
prevent this being a hit of
offensive magnitude, I
suppose.

Abandoning ambitions to become a vet, Newton-John's debut single had been released way back in 1966, before a fleeting spell in Monkee-styled *Toomorrow* and a failed attempt to win the Eurovision song contest for England (her country of birth). For a period, she was America's best-selling country star and had even released her own *Greatest Hits* package earlier in 1978, which had reached No. 19 in the UK album charts.

Carr first met Olivia Newton-John at a dinner party. The latter only agreed to take on the role of Sandy in *Grease* because the film was to be a musical. Newton-John's own musical director, John Farrar, was invited to pen some tunes for the film and came up with the songs 'Hopelessly Devoted To You' and 'You're The One . . .', the latter an electrifying stomp of a finale.

For this last sequence, Sandy's image of virginal naiveté – complete with immaculately combed and flicked hair-do, circular skirt and pastel-coloured cardigan – is cast off in exchange for a leather-clad, shoulder-revealing, stiletto-heeled vamp who turns the table on Travolta's previously cocksure character.

'You're The One That I Want' was the big smash single of 1978, itself a record year for vinyl sales. It stayed at the top of the charts for nine weeks, sold two million copies in the US alone and successfully kept The Smurfs off the No. 1 slot for six consecutive weeks. The soundtrack album was No. 1 in both America and the UK for three months.

> 'John Farrar was invited to pen some tunes for the film and came up with the songs "Hopelessly Devoted To You" and "You're The One . . .", the latter an electrifying stomp of a finale.'

Also in this year . . .

* Keith Moon died at his Mayfair flat after an overdose of Heminevrin.
* The Police enjoyed their first singles success with 'Can't Stand Losing You' and 'Roxanne'.
* The Jam began to receive critical acclaim for their original and incendiary live shows.
* Dire Straits lifted themselves out of the low-key London pub circuit and signed a recording contract that would eventually turn them into one of the world's biggest acts.
* The Clash headlined a huge Rock Against Racism gig in central London.

THRILLS

FEVER!

THE RECEPTION

AFTER THE BOOK, the play . . . after the film, the obscenity.

I've been to a few record company parties, average creep quotient 80 per cent, and they are usually glib self-congratulatory affairs, but I usually figure if I've bought their records in the past they at least owe me a few rounds. However, the reception after the premiere of *Grease* made even the largest do I'd previously been to look like the pie stall at Waterloo.

The Lyceum ballroom in the Strand had been specially hired for the night, and the police were shoving back hordes of teenage Travolta-ites outside who were watching in awe as Rollo alter Rollo delivered m'lords, ladies and 'celebrities' onto the red carpet.

"While the poor people sleeping with the shade on the light? While the poor people sleeping all the stars come out as night."

Inside the place was made up like a royal wedding. Red velvet tables with candles, very long tables attended by hordes of high-hatted chefs, decked out with hogs heads with apples in their mouths, sides of beef, large sheep's tongues, hams, unpronounceable French dishes, assorted salads, cheeses and fruits. Legions of waitresses, who were bawled out if not prompt, always ready with more brandy or wine (I'm sure it was an excellent year).

And of course champagne, champagne, champagne.

Trying to bring a little L.A. to London, young dents in Newton-John outfits squeaked and lisped, skweezdiung-nktevon to "sticky" or "Francoise" or "Zoe," acting ridiculously 'effervescent' on the dance floor in attempts to show how 'rebellious' and 'free' one can get.

Their male counterparts, obviously aware that the man himself hung large over the night, went through some outlandish gyrations as if always on the verge of going into some substantial dance steps whereas they were just hoping to fool the casual onlooker. As usual, this sad strain of over-thirties were in their pointed collar shirts slashed to the waist (revealing the obligatory medallion and disgusting grey-haired chests), and tight-arsed flairs.

At a table behind me, a group of long-haired men who may well have been one of those Bad Company or Foreigner type groups, asked one of the young servants to bring them one of the large chocolate gateaux cakes from the other side of the hall. After she'd struggled back with it, the group proceeded to squash their hands in it and then try and wipe it on each other.

It seemed everyone knew each other — a kind of decadent twilight society that gathers in exclusive clubs and parties to shut off the world and cling to each other, desperately attempting to retain the old orders and wealth. Old men dribbling through alcohole conversations with their young girl friends, women getting snotty and rude with the bar staff and waitresses, the whole mass slowly collapsing in its wretched drunkenness.

This is no working class bigotry on my part. This obscene affair, costing countless thousands, had come the night after BBC's documentary on the poverty in which the homes for handicapped children find themselves.

You may find that clichéd, but if you want to sneer cynically over things like this, I'll break your skull. Promise.

Celebrities included Russell Harty, Liew Gardener and the awful Susan George (who was obviously speeding badly). More may have showed (wisely Travolta didn't), I left after

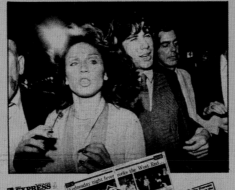

fifty minutes. Outside young girls were still waiting.

"Oi mista, get us in!" two shouted at me. I took my invite from my inside pocket and handed it to one of them —after all, she had probably bought the album and the book and would queue to see the film soon. Stunned at her bluff being called, she just looked at it a while and then handed it back.

"Nah, leave it out," she said. "They wouldn't let us in there . . ." Ain't that the truth.

DANNY BAKER

THE PHENOMENON

IT WAS EVERY News Editor's dream: a genuine shock-horror week.

The Liberal party, already reeling from the serious charges against their former leader Jeremy Thorpe, were further rocked by allegations of sex offences at the National Liberal Club. Both recent Labour and Conservative governments seemed likely to be implicated in the Rhodesian sanctions-busting scandal. A Bulgarian defector was murdered at the Aldwych with a lethal umbrella. Cases of smallpox, typhoid and lassa fever were making horrifying reading. And in Persia the Shit Of Iran was attending to business with what was, even by his standards, rare vigour, massacring thousands of peasants.

With such a cornucopia of sensation to select from, which item did the best-selling national dailies choose as their lead story last Thursday?

That's right — John Travolta.

In their reports of the scenes outside the Empire at the premiere of *Grease*, the papers were single-minded: "FIGHT FEVER" (*Daily Mirror*); "GREASE FEVER" (*Daily Express*); "TRAVOLTA FEVER" (*The Sun* — characteristically bereft of even a modicum of originality; that headline had been used by *The Observer* in March and *Time* in April.)

The only one of the tabloids to give preference to politics, the *Daily Mail*, made up for lost column inches by devoting most of pages two and three to the story. Even *The Times* deemed it necessary to include a short report ("Women faint for John Travolta").

Although the recent *Gusbag* correspondent who suggested that the only difference between *NME* and the *Daily Mirror* was 11p could have made reference to *NME*'s superior journalism as a further distinguishing factor, the accuracy of his observation was clearly demonstrated — the popular press seem to be taking their 'pop' coverage ever more seriously.

Certainly the hysterical reaction of the press paralleled that of the 5,000 fans. Describing the occasion as "a riot," David Wigg wrote in the *Daily Express*: "London has seen nothing like it since Beatlemania," while a policeman quoted in *The Sun* went further: "I have been on duty in the days of Beatlemania and The Rolling Stones — but I've never seen anything like this."

Strange perhaps, considering that Travolta's appeal must be based solely on his Saturday *Night Fever* performance. (Although it should be remembered that Beatlemania, on a national scale, was also a spontaneous phenomenon). The *Mail* had its own explanation: "The film company had organised a massive publicity campaign. This was the sixth international premiere and there have been violent incidents at others."

However, the size of the crowd in Leicester Square cannot be explained simply by hyper-efficient PR, nor even by the fact that no film has ever previously had the benefit of a nine-week chart-topping single as advance publicity.

Travolta clearly has an individual charisma which beggars literal description or analysis, and this has been evident for some time. In its Travolta cover story last March, *The Observer Colour Magazine* said: "For the past two years he has been a U.S. teenage idol on a scale that is unimaginable in this country." Jane Fonda asked him what it was like to be a real star

● *Continues next page*

● *Continues next page*

Lone Groover Fever   BENYON

"Y'KNOW, ITS ONLY BIN ILLEGAL T'SMOKE DOPE FOR 50 YEARS — THAT'S WHEN THEY BROUGHT TH' LAW OUT!"

"THOSE WERE TH' 20'S, PRONTO WE WERE ON TH' BRINK OF A WORKERS' REVOLUTION"

"THAT'S WHY THEY CALL THOSE YEARS TH' DEPRESSION"

"THEY KEPT EVERYONE OFF GRASS . . . ALL THEY COULD GET WERE DOWNERS —"

"HENCE, NO REVOLTO"

"HENCE STATUS QUO!"

7

Relax
Frankie Goes To Hollywood

Release Date: 26.11.83
No. Weeks In Chart: 59
Reached No. 1: 28.01.84
Total Sales: 1,910,000

Arguably one of the most controversial singles ever released, 'Relax' was an overtly sexual blast, announcing the unknown Frankie Goes To Hollywood as the country's biggest – and most shocking – band.

The seedy beast that was Frankie crawled out from the cauldron of talent swirling around Eric's club in Liverpool, an early stomping ground for numerous stars, including Echo and the Bunnymen, KLF, Pete Burns and the Lightning Seeds' Ian Broudie. Sudanese-born frontman Holly Johnson enjoyed a fleeting success alongside Bill Drummond and Ian Broudie with Big In Japan, an outfit with few releases but widespread acclaim, but left after two country-influenced singles.

Johnson was left to lick his wounds and retire to the shadows, where he formulated his masterplan while working as a labourer and pizza chef. After a couple of low-profile solo singles, which he dubbed 'cowboy sleaze', Johnson recruited Nasher Nash, Mark O'Toole, Peter Gill and female vocalist Sonya Mazunda following a chance meeting in a record store. Taking their moniker from a newspaper clipping about either Frank Sinatra or Frankie

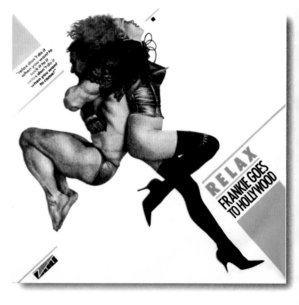

Vaughan (the band would never say which), Frankie Goes To Hollywood was born. One night, Johnson walked in late to a rehearsal at

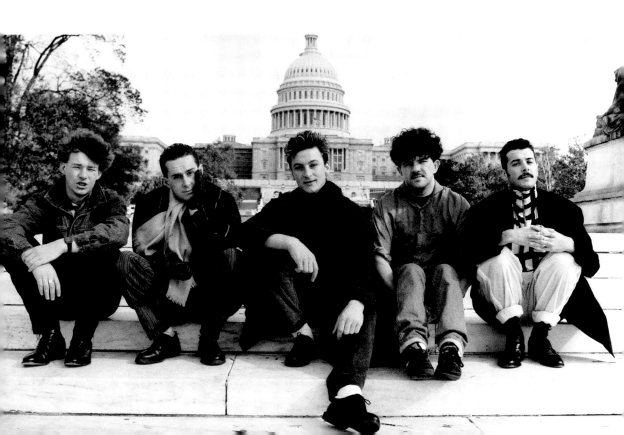

an old police cell and caught the band jamming along feverishly to a single, repetitive, but booming bass note. He started to improvise the lyrics and so 'Relax' was born. At their debut gig in a Liverpool pub, Clash fan and former Opium Eaters and Spitfire Boys member Paul Rutherford climbed on stage and effectively 'joined' the band at the expense of Sonya.

The early years were quiet for Frankie, playing the rounds of the S&M/gay cabaret scene, sporting their buttock-revealing leather bondage gear. Major record labels winced at their musical and lyrical content – perhaps the self-proclaimed tag of 'post-punk S&M gay cabaret act' didn't help. Then former Bubbles musician and noted producer Trevor Horn saw them on the television show *The Tube* (for which he had written the theme tune) and promptly signed the band to his ZTT label, home also to the noise terrorists, Art of Noise and Propaganda.

History tells us that it wasn't until DJ Mike Read banned 'Relax' that it hit the top spot. Actually, Read simply objected to the sexual lyrics and pulled the vinyl off mid-track – the

BBC took the formal step of banning the record (and the accompanying video). With hindsight, this was a little odd as station stalwarts John Peel and Kid Jensen had both invited the Liverpudlian trouble-makers to record Radio One sessions a full year before the eventual censorship – and those studio appearances had included this now contraband track, 'Relax', which had been played more than a dozen times previously on the national radio. Stories about the use of session musicians and veterans from Ian Dury's The Blockheads for the studio recording of 'Relax' did little to dampen Frankie's appeal. Perhaps this was because the debut single was such a staggering track, and sounded like nothing that had gone before. Add to this the subsequent radio ban, the suggestive graphics and sexual lyrics, and ZTT and Frankie had a pop music time bomb on their hands.

Initially, the single had charted at No. 77. But after the radio opposition it shot to No. 1, where it stayed for five weeks, remaining in the charts for one entire year ('Gay Sex Tops Pops' as one tabloid put it). Complemented by vast sales of their 'Frankie Says' monochrome T-shirts – which, incidentally, were subject to mass piracy yet still broke all official band-merchandise records – and a strikingly militaristic logo, the five-piece from Liverpool were the masters of 1984. Total sales edged near to two million copies when 'Relax' enjoyed a resurgence on the release of the equally staggering follow-up single, 'Two Tribes'. 'Relax' just never dates, and remains a simple, brash and crunching musical behemoth that was, and still is, quite breathtaking.

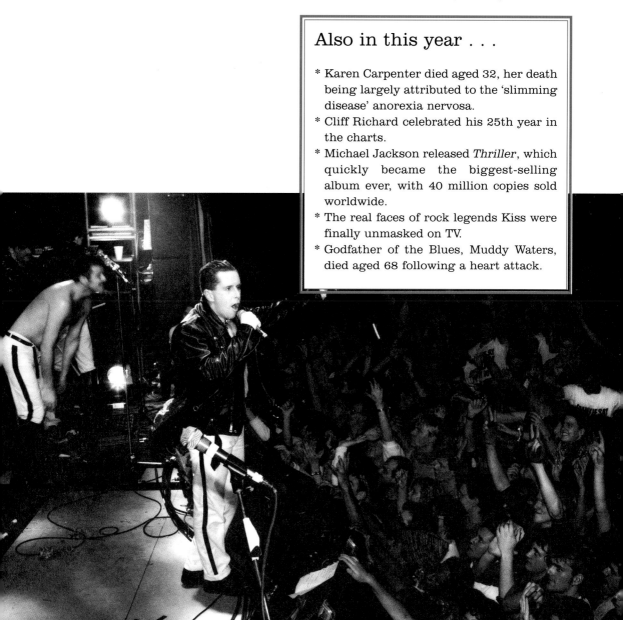

Also in this year . . .

* Karen Carpenter died aged 32, her death being largely attributed to the 'slimming disease' anorexia nervosa.
* Cliff Richard celebrated his 25th year in the charts.
* Michael Jackson released *Thriller*, which quickly became the biggest-selling album ever, with 40 million copies sold worldwide.
* The real faces of rock legends Kiss were finally unmasked on TV.
* Godfather of the Blues, Muddy Waters, died aged 68 following a heart attack.

8

She Loves You
The Beatles

Release Date: 29.08.63
No. Weeks In Chart: 36
Reached No. 1: 12.09.63
Total Sales: 1,890,000

This highly infectious slab of pop genius is the best-selling Beatles hit in the UK, the song that created Beatlemania and changed everything, forever.

It is hard to imagine a time when The Beatles were not the most famous band in the world. Their debut single, 'Love Me Do', had pierced the Top 20 and further excellent progress had been made by the No. 2 'Please Please Me' and then by their first No. 1 hit, 'From Me To You'. However, relative to their latterday status as living legends, The Beatles who released 'She Loves You' were mere novices.

The year 1963 had started inauspiciously enough with their first headline tour around Scotland, where they were still considered obscure enough to require a billing as 'The Love Me Do Boys'. The former Silver Beetles' first nationwide tour was even followed by a school gig for £100 at the request of a pupil at Stowe School, in Buckinghamshire; they played at the school's own Roxburgh Hall.

However, September 1963's 'She Loves You' opened the floodgates of Beatlemania and started to ink The Beatles' indelible mark on twentieth-century culture. A series of high-profile events served to swell momentum behind the Fab Four – their first live TV show won huge

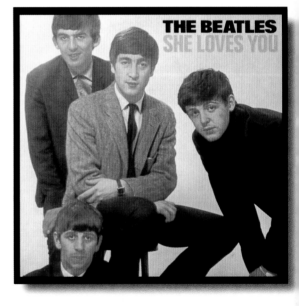

ratings, then a top-of-the-bill performance at *Sunday Night at the Palladium* introduced them into the nation's living rooms. Following this (mimed) appearance, the newspaper headlines declared that Beatlemania had arrived.

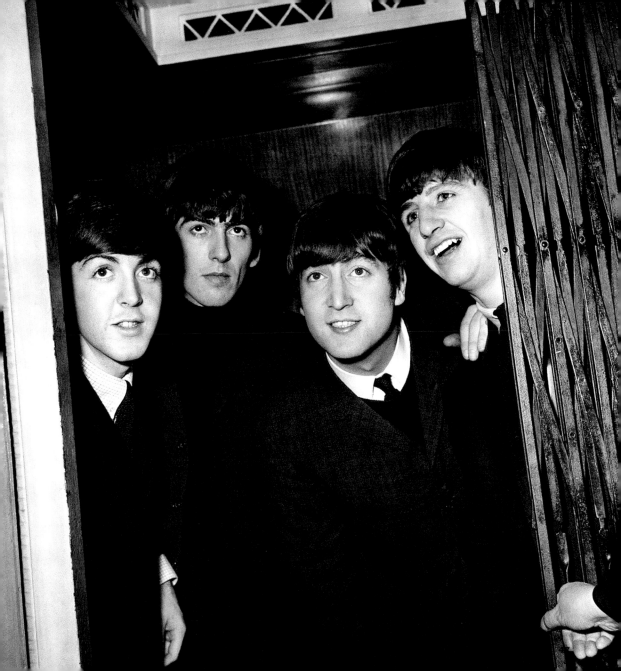

NME TOP THIRTY

(Wednesday, September 4, 1963)

Last This
Week

2 1	SHE LOVES YOU
	Beatles (Parlophone)
1 2	BAD TO ME
	Billy J. Kramer (Parlophone)
3 3	I'M TELLIN' YOU NOW
	Freddie and the Dreamers
	(Columbia)
4 4	IT'S ALL IN THE GAME
	Cliff Richard (Columbia)
6 5	I'LL NEVER GET OVER YOU
	Johnny Kidd (HMV)
7 6	YOU DON'T HAVE TO BE
	A BABY TO CRY
	Caravelles (Decca-Ritz)
10 7	I WANT TO STAY HERE
	Steve Lawrence-Eydie Gorme
	(CBS)
13 8	JUST LIKE EDDIE
	Heinz (Decca)
5 8	SWEETS FOR MY SWEET
	Searchers (Pye)
9 10	THE LEGION'S LAST
	PATROL Ken Thorne (HMV)
8 11	WIPE OUT
	Surfaris (London)
12 12	IN SUMMER
	Billy Fury (Decca)
10 13	TWIST AND SHOUT (EP)
	Beatles (Parlophone)
16 14	DANCE ON
	Kathy Kirby (Decca)
14 15	I'M CONFESSIN'
	Frank Ifield (Columbia)
24 16	I WANT TO STAY HERE
	Miki and Griff (Pye)
17 17	STILL Karl Denver (Decca)
27 18	WHISPERING
	Bachelors (Decca)
— 19	APPLEJACK
	Jet Harris-Tony Meehan
	(Decca)
— 20	STILL Ken Dodd (Columbia)
15 21	TWIST AND SHOUT
	Brian Poole and the
	Tremeloes (Decca)
20 22	TWO SILHOUETTES
	Del Shannon (London)
25 22	COME ON
	Rolling Stones (Decca)
— 24	FRANKIE AND JOHNNY
	Sam Cooke (RCA)
30 25	SURF CITY
	Jan & Dean (Liberty)
— 26	WISHING
	Buddy Holly (Coral)
19 27	THE CRUEL SEA
	Dakotas (Parlophone)
21 28	DEVIL IN DISGUISE
	Elvis Presley (RCA)
29 29	ACAPULCO 1922
	Kenny Ball (Pye)
18 30	SUKIYAKI
	Kyu Sakamoto (HMV)

BEST SELLING POP RECORDS IN U.S.

by courtesy of "Billboard"

Last This (Tuesday, Sept. 3, 1963)
Week

1 1	MY BOYFRIEND'S BACK
	Angels
2 2	HELLO MUDDUH, HELLO
	FADDUH Allan Sherman
6 3	IF I HAD A HAMMER
	Trini Lopez
11 4	BLUE VELVET Bobby Vinton
4 5	CANDY GIRL Four Seasons
10 6	HEAT WAVE
	Martha and the Vandellas
8 7	MOCKINGBIRD Inez Foxx
12 8	THE MONKEY TIME
	Major Lance
5 9	BLOWIN' IN THE WIND
	Peter, Paul and Mary
15 10	HEY GIRL Freddie Scott
3 11	FINGERTIPS
	Little Stevie Wonder
13 12	SURFER GIRL Beach Boys
10 13	DENISE Randy & the Rainbows
19 14	FRANKIE AND JOHNNY
	Sam Cooke
20 15	THEN HE KISSED ME Crystals
16 16	DANKE SCHOEN Wayne Newton
9 17	MORE Kai Winding
7 18	JUDY'S TURN TO CRY
	Lesley Gore
— 19	YOU CAN NEVER STOP ME
	LOVING YOU Johnny Tillotson
— 20	PAINTED, TAINTED ROSE
	Al Martino

BEST SELLING SHEET MUSIC IN BRITAIN

Last This (Tuesday, Sept. 3, 1963)
Week

2 1	I'M TELLIN' YOU NOW
	(Feldman)
1 2	BAD TO ME (Northern Songs)
13 3	SHE LOVES YOU
	(Northern Songs)
6 4	I'LL NEVER GET OVER YOU
	(Leeds)
4 5	IT'S ALL IN THE GAME
	(Blossom)
6 6	THE LEGION'S LAST PATROL
	(Filmusic)
3 7	SWEETS FOR MY SWEET
	(Hill and Range)
7 8	TWIST AND SHOUT (Belinda)
9 9	THE CRUEL SEA (Jarp)
4 10	I'M CONFESSIN'
	(Francis, Day and Hunter)
8 11	IN SUMMER (Skidmore)
14 12	ACAPULCO 1922 (Burlington)
12 13	WIPE OUT (Ambassador)
13 14	ATLANTIS
	(Francis, Day and Hunter)
11 15	WELCOME TO MY WORLD
	(142 Music)
20 16	YOU DON'T HAVE TO BE A
	BABY TO CRY (Frank)
9 17	TAKE THESE CHAINS FROM
	MY HEART (Acuff-Rose)
25 18	IF I RULED THE WORLD
	(Sterling)
— 19	I WANT TO STAY HERE
	(Aldon)
21 20	I LIKE IT (Jarp)
19 21	SUKIYAKI (Welbeck-Hozi)
22 22	STILL (Peter Maurice)
17 23	YOU CAN NEVER STOP ME
	LOVING YOU (Cramer)
22 24	THE GOOD LIFE (World Wide)
26 25	JUST LIKE EDDIE (Meridian)
18 26	DEVIL IN DISGUISE (West One)
22 27	NOBODY'S DARLIN' BUT
	MINE (Peter Maurice)
— 28	IF YOU GOTTA MAKE A FOOL
	OF SOMEBODY (Feldman)
— 29	IT'S TOO LATE NOW (Romney)
— 30	HOW DO YOU DO IT
	(Dick James)
— 30	THOSE LAZY-HAZY-CRAZY
	DAYS OF SUMMER (Comet)

Also in this year . . .

* Country music star Patsy Cline was killed when the aircraft in which she was flying crashed in Tennessee, USA.
* Bob Dylan's debut album sold an initial 5,000 copies.
* Buddy Holly enjoyed three posthumous hit songs, ending with 'Wishin'' in September of 1963.
* Phil Spector withdrew his seasonal *meisterwork*, 'A Christmas Gift To You', out of respect for the assassinated US President, John F Kennedy.
* Edith Piaf, France's most popular singer, died at the age of 48.

The discursive dynamic of the lyrics was considered unusual at the time. Lennon and McCartney were said to have penned the melody and lyrics while sitting opposite each other, staring eye to eye.

This song was the second in a record eleven consecutive No. 1 hits for The Beatles. Of the 1.89 million sales it has made, 85 per cent came in advance orders. Such was its popularity that it returned to the No. 1 spot in late November of 1963, just over two months after it had first hit the top slot – at a time when their debut album *Please Please Me* had just been usurped at the top of the long-player charts by its follow-up, *With The Beatles*.

This song's chart career did not finish there, either – 'She Loves You' re-charted in April 1964

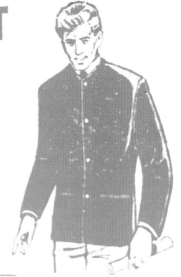
(buoyed by their US chart success) and then, nearly twenty years later, and off the back of a batch of re-releases, it re-charted yet again in 1983. It remained the best-selling single in UK chart history for another 24 years, until Paul McCartney's band Wings stole that crown with 'Mull of Kintyre' (see No. 4).

Within a few short months, the close harmonies, catchy guitar riffs, fashionable clothes and parent-baiting haircuts had made The Beatles the most talked-about band on the planet. The seedy strip joints and Liverpool nightclubs where they had been performing twice a night less than a year previously now seemed a million miles away.

Interestingly, the five entries for The Beatles in this list are all within 28 months of one other, and are also from the 'early' period, when Beatlemania was at its peak. Although later releases were considered perhaps more sophisticated and critically praiseworthy, it is this batch of early to mid-'60s' releases that secured the band's place in history.

'She Loves You' was a moment of magic, which came long before Beatles' gigs became unbearable due to the ear-splitting din of fans' screaming, before the long-haired four travelled the globe in search of spiritual retreats, before their much-publicised drug experimentation, inter-band quarrelling and the eventual rupture in 1970.

In short, this song was a pop watershed by which all future singles must be judged. Pure, unadulterated pop genius.

9

Unchained Melody/(There'll Be Blue-birds Over) The White Cliffs of Dover
Robson Green and Jerome Flynn

Release Date: 20.05.95
No. Weeks In Chart: 17
Reached No. 1: 20.05.95
Total Sales: 1,843,701

By the end of 1995, 'Unchained Melody' had become the biggest-selling single since Band Aid's stupendous 1984 hit 'Do They Know It's Christmas?'

This song is the biggest-selling single ever released by an act whose primary profession was not music. The staggering sales statistics of Robson Green and Jerome Flynn prove the indisputable power of terrestrial television coverage, a benefit felt by many of the records in this list. Both men were actors who had come to the music industry thanks to the huge popularity of their first major lead roles in the period piece and ratings winner, *Soldier, Soldier*.

In one episode of this successful TV drama, Robson and Jerome's respective characters sang 'Unchained Melody' at an army talent contest, following the screening of which the broadcaster's switchboard received a record number of enquiries.

Enter Simon Cowell, latterly of *Pop Idol* fame and *übermeister* of numerous pop careers, including Westlife and Gareth Gates. After tracking down Robson and Jerome's acting agent, he was told that they were not interested in releasing a record. Cowell persevered and even contacted Robson's mother to help

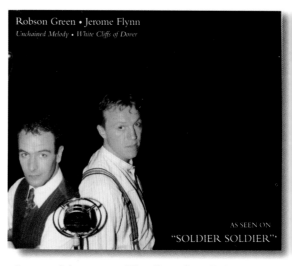

Robson Green • Jerome Flynn
Unchained Melody • White Cliffs of Dover

AS SEEN ON
"SOLDIER SOLDIER"

advance his cause. Finally, after Robson had faxed nature-loving Jerome – who was on a back-to-his-roots pilgrimage in the mountains at the time – a deal was struck.

The subsequent avalanche of advance orders took even the seasoned Cowell by surprise. First-week sales reached 310,000, ensuring a new entry at No. 1. The next week, sales rose by

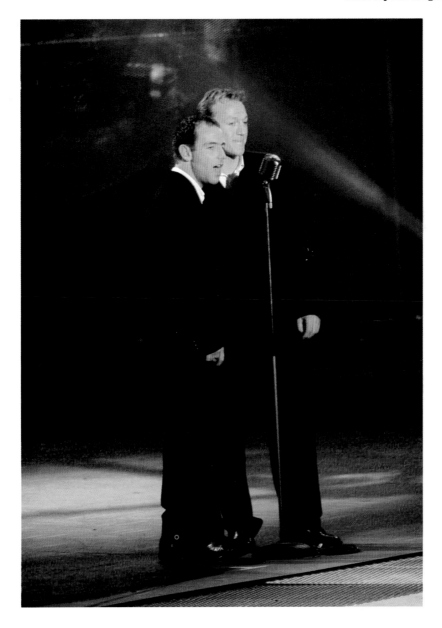

nearly 50 per cent to 460,000. The following week, the duo went triple platinum with one million sales. The song was a commercial juggernaut. Admirably, the single also generated over £30,000 towards the charity Greenpeace's coffers.

A blond-haired, blue-eyed Jerome Flynn was born in the Kent countryside into a family of modest means, and was one of three children. He showed an artistic flair at an early age, and was soon acting in local amateur dramatics and school productions, including *The Crucible*, directed by his brother Daniel. He was also in a school band named System X, which was booed off stage when they started playing Stranglers' hits to a crowd of old-aged pensioners.

Abandoning his A-level studies in exchange for life at the Central School of Speech and Drama, in London's Swiss Cottage, Jerome's acting career gradually progressed (peppered with numerous travels abroad) and he even enjoyed a short stint in a group with the name of Carte Blanche.

After qualifying for Equity membership he progressed still further, until he landed the role in *Soldier, Soldier*. It was in this show that he co-starred with Geordie Robson Golightly Green, also one of three children, although from almost the opposite end of the country.

Born in a small mining village just outside Newcastle upon Tyne and a year younger than Jerome, Green – the son of a miner – had dreamed initially of becoming a RAF pilot. School productions, including *Joseph and the Amazing Technicolour Dreamcoat*, set him off on the path of acting, however, whereby he later joined various amateur dramatic societies, as well as forming his own band, Solid State.

After leaving school, Green signed up to become an apprentice draughtsman at a shipbuilders in North Tyneside – yet after qualifying, he bravely changed career direction in order to enrol with Newcastle's Live Theatre. Tours around the north-east followed, before his television break came – ironically, in a drama about coalminers. He then played various minor roles before winning the part of hospital porter Jimmy in the medical drama *Casualty*. Like Jerome, *Soldier, Soldier* was also his first co-starring role.

Following the duo's surprising single success, two further singles were released (see No. 63), as well as a hugely popular album.

Also in this year . . .

* R.E.M. drummer Bill Berry suffered a brain aneurysm while performing on stage in Switzerland.
* Take That notched up their penultimate and seventh No. 1 hit with 'Never Forget.' A year later, they split up.
* *The Beatles Anthology 1* was the year's biggest-selling album.
* Michael Jackson sailed a 50-foot statue of himself down the River Thames in London, as part of his promotional campaign for his *HIStory* double album.
* Blur battled Oasis for the No. 1 single spot as Britpop took over the charts.

'The staggering sales statistics of Robson Green and Jerome Flynn prove the indisputable power of terrestrial television coverage.'

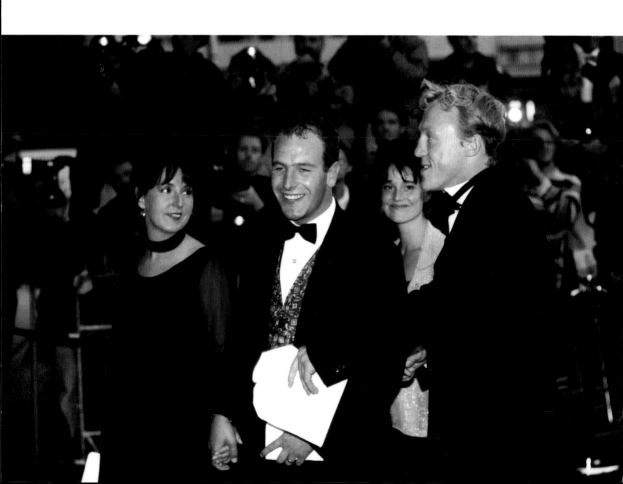

10 Mary's Boy Child/Oh My Lord
Boney M

Release Date:	2.12.78
No. Weeks In Chart:	8
Reached No. 1:	9.12.78
Total Sales:	1,790,000

By the time Boney M came onto the scene, many underground disco fans were already recoiling from the apparent mainstream hijacking of their genre.

Part of Boney M's attraction was that they seemed oblivious to the bared teeth of punk, the barbed pens of their media critics or, indeed, most commercial sales records. They completed their brace of UK No. 1 singles with this festive hit, a tune that was originally a hit for Harry Belafonte in 1957 (see No. 51). Unfortunately, they were to have only one other Top Five hit (the sing-a-long of 'Hooray! Hooray! It's a Holi-Holiday') before their chart positions slid away as quickly as disco became an anachronism.

'Disco' was initially a term used to refer to the action of dancing to a record rather than to a live band, which had been the norm prior to the onset of disco fever. Some trace disco back as far as 1968, and to Sly and the Family Stone's 'Dance To The Music'. Others point to elements of James Brown and early Isaac Hayes or the Ojays' 'Love Train'. Early disco clubs sprang up in 1974 on America's West Coast, but the tradition was taken to its logical, high-profile extreme by New York's super-club, Studio 54.

Of course, what sent disco overground was the white flared suit and street-strutting style of John Travolta in the blockbuster 1978 film *Saturday Night Fever*, with its corresponding record-breaking soundtrack courtesy of the shrill falsetto of The Bee Gees.

Boney M never enjoyed the critical acclaim of artists such as Gloria Gaynor, Chic and Donna Summer (whose 'I Feel Love' is often credited with inventing techno music), yet none of these

A Boney Xmas!

IT LOOKS AS though Boney M (currently leading the NME Chart Points Table for 1978, though being closely challenged by Travolta & Newton-John) will have this year's big Christmas hit single. They've just recorded their version of "Mary's Boy Child", Belafonte's 1957 hit, for November 24 release by Atlantic-Hansa.

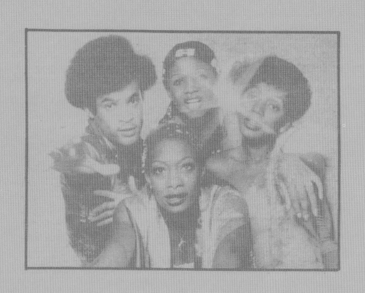

artists feature in this list. Meanwhile, American society never quite got over the shock of discovering that The Village People were not just a mixed-race workers' union; but by then, the emergence of the gay scene that had nurtured disco from its very beginning had had a seismic effect on homosexual and civil rights and other social issues.

Disco's death knell – and thus the beginning of the end for Boney M – came with the 'Disco Sucks' campaign in the US, when thousands of people burned their most-hated disco records during halftime of a football game. Disco hits for rock acts such as Rod Stewart and even The Rolling Stones killed its street cool. Although Boney M had only the one hit in the US (see No. 5), this opposition together with the changing tides of British music – punk, early Two Tone, Gary Numan – put the writing on the wall. This was despite the fact that sales figures of such genres were dwarfed by Boney M's historically notable achievements.

This version of the song remains the biggest-selling medley of all time, combining as it does the tune originally sung by Harry Belafonte way back in 1957 (see No. 51 – this was one of the first sensational million-sellers) and 'Oh My Lord', written by Frank Farian.

By 1980, Boney M's big hits had dried up, and shortly after the band split up. They reformed in 1989, although at one point there were three different versions of the band touring simultaneously. Occasional so-called 'Mega-mixes' of their classic hits still sell in sizeable quantities. Frank Farian came back to public prominence in the late '80s, when he was revealed to be the man behind Milli Vanilli, whose singing exploits – or rather lack of – caused outrage in the music industry.

Nonetheless, despite the sense that their image at least, if not their music, will always be a time-piece, Boney M's eighteen Platinum and fifteen Gold discs for albums, plus over 200 Gold and Platinum discs for hit singles, with in excess of 150 million global sales, signifies an indelible mark on music history that cannot be denied.

One other achievement must be theirs – the oddest album title ever: *Boonoonoonoos*.

Also in this year . . .

* Boomtown Rats enjoyed their first of two No. 1 hits with 'Ratrap'.
* Critically acclaimed Patti Smith enjoyed a hit single with 'Because The Night', co-written by Bruce Springsteen.
* *Saturday Night Fever* was a smash box-office hit and revitalised the career of the Bee Gees.
* New York band Talking Heads began to make waves on the UK underground.
* New York's most famous disco dance floor, Studio 54, was busted by narcotics officers working undercover as drug dealers.
* Meatloaf introduced the world to his unique talent with 'You Took The Words Right Out Of My Mouth'.

THRILLS

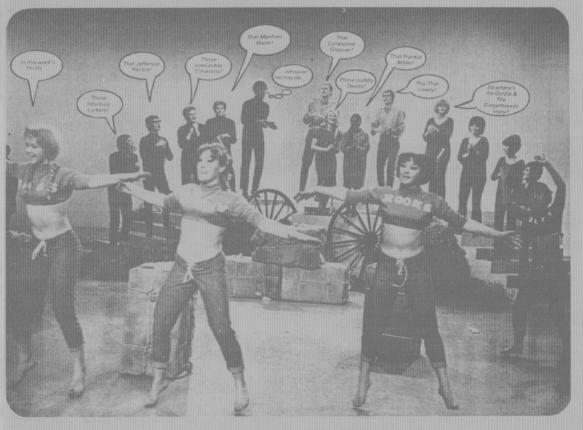

DISCO TAKES OVER ENTIRE UNIVERSE!

11 Love Is All Around
Wet Wet Wet

Release Date: 21.05.94
No. Weeks In Chart: 37
Reached No. 1: 4.06.94
Total Sales: 1,783,827

The band became so concerned about the possible suffocating effects of the colossal sales and over-exposure of this single, that their manager was reported to have phoned from abroad to insist on the song being deleted.

This soul-pop outfit made up of Glaswegian school friends enjoyed their third and final UK No. 1 with a cover of the 1967 Top Five Troggs' song. Lead singer Marti Pellow's striking good looks and soulful voice, plus the band's technical ability, gave them a convincing blend of musical credibility and teenage adoration – a powerful chemistry.

Supposedly chased by most major record companies after just one demo tape had been farmed out, the band's debut was the Top Ten feel-good pop of 'Wishing I Was Lucky'. 'Love Is All Around' was taken from the British box-office smash film, *Four Weddings and a Funeral*. The movie followed the turbulent love life of a bumbling serial monogamist, perfectly played by Hugh Grant, and its huge popularity ensured the single's place as the longest-reigning No. 1 by a British act.

Pellow's constantly chirpy demeanour and seemingly permanent smile masked a serious drug addiction that he eventually went public

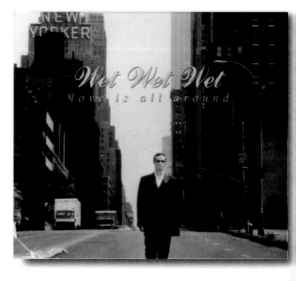

with, before forging a modest solo career, which included a critically lauded run in the West End show *Chicago*. The Troggs' Reg Presley declared he would be spending the massive royalties on studying crop circles.

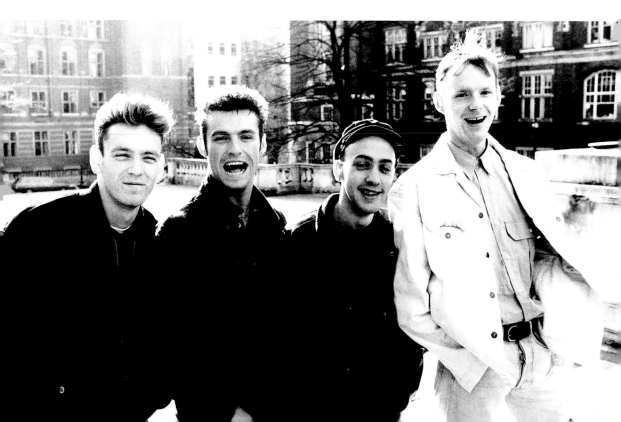

12 Anything Is Possible/Evergreen
Will Young

Release Date: 9.03.02
No. Weeks In Chart: 16
Reached No. 1: 9.03.02
Total Sales: 1,779,938

This is the biggest-selling single since Elton John's 'Candle In The Wind 97' and the commercial culmination of the cultural phenomenon that is the 'reality' audition TV show.

Will Young triumphed over 10,000 other pop wannabes in the race to become Britain's first Pop Idol. Although the very last person to be accepted for the final auditions, this 23-year-old politics graduate began to win supporters after he famously confronted the villainous judge, Simon Cowell, live on air.

Seen as the 'posh' contestant, Young joked about how, in response to Cowell's barbs, his father would be likely to say to his mother, 'Get the shot gun, Annabel.' He was always second favourite, behind teen heart-throb Gareth Gates (see No. 38), and seemed as shocked as the rest of the nation was by his dramatic win. Young polled 4.6 million votes over Gates' 4.1 million – jointly, more than the number won by the Conservative Party at the 2001 election.

Young, a non-identical twin, had been in a TV boy band, winning through to the final line-up of a GMTV outfit, but had had no significant success. Perhaps this song was not the best showcase for his sophisticated vocal range, which Pete Waterman described as the 'best voice I've heard in twenty years'. It mattered

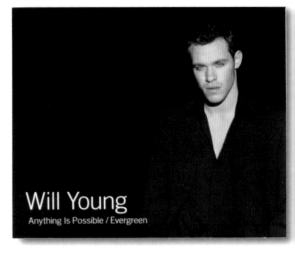

little to the fans, who bought the single in record-breaking quantities. Following his win, and despite industry concerns about his career and fanbase, Young announced that he was gay.

Outside his singing career, Young has also appeared on the catwalk, done occasional photographic work, worked in bars and even been a personal assistant at Sony Music.

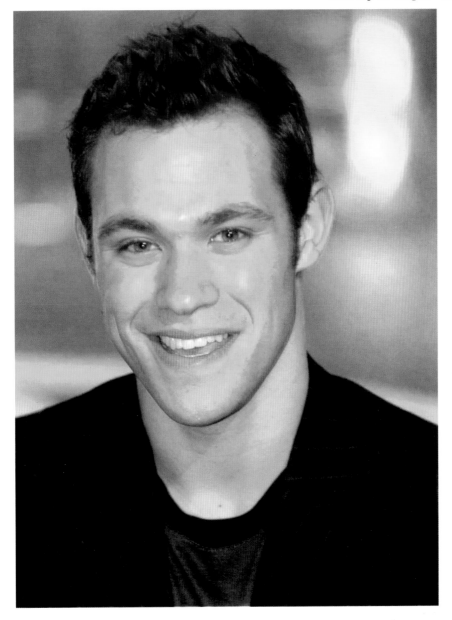

13 I Just Called To Say I Loved You
Stevie Wonder

Release Date: 25.08.84
No. Weeks In Chart: 26
Reached No. 1: 8.09.84
Total Sales: 1,775,000

This song is not generally regarded as Wonder's creative pinnacle – his other, more pioneering pieces are heavily sampled and acutely influential, and he is regarded as one of the prime movers in progressing and pushing back the boundaries of soul and R&B.

This is Wonder's only solo No. 1 and Motown's biggest-ever UK single – in any other year, its 1.77 million sales would have been unsurpassed; but this was not allowing for Bob Geldof (see No. 2). Paradoxically, Wonder has received gushing critical acclaim for his early '70s' work, including the seminal albums *Talking Book* (with its title in braille on the album cover) and *Songs in the Key of Life*, yet he enjoyed his greatest UK chart success during the early '80s.

This track was taken from the Oscar-winning soundtrack to the movie *Woman In Red*, which starred Gene Wilder. The song replaced George Michael's 'Careless Whisper' at No.1, giving the charts three million sellers in a row at the top (see No.'s 22 and 34).

Blinded by the effects of too much oxygen in an incubator shortly after his birth, Wonder would also lose his sense of smell after a serious car crash in 1973, which left him in a coma for four days. A child prodigy, he was a multi-instrumentalist at the age of seven, a songwriter at the age of eight and signed to Motown aged ten as Little Stevie Wonder.

His flop debut single, 'I Call It Pretty Music But The Old People Call It The Blues', had then-session drummer Marvin Gaye in the studio; by a curious twist of fate, this 1984 transatlantic No. 1 came just months after Gaye had been shot dead. Two months later, Wonder could be heard playing the harmonica on Chaka Khan's own No. 1 hit, 'I Feel For You'.

Stevie Wonder is also renowned for having campaigned successfully to turn US civil rights campaigner Martin Luther King's birthday into an American National Holiday. Wonder is also a prolific songwriter for other recording artists, including co-writing 'The Tears of a Clown' with Smokey Robinson.

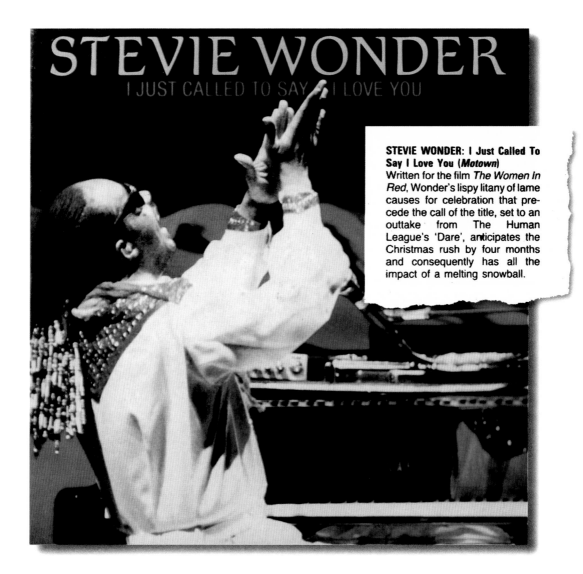

STEVIE WONDER: I Just Called To Say I Love You (*Motown*)
Written for the film *The Women In Red*, Wonder's lispy litany of lame causes for celebration that precede the call of the title, set to an outtake from The Human League's 'Dare', anticipates the Christmas rush by four months and consequently has all the impact of a melting snowball.

14

I Want To Hold Your Hand
The Beatles

Release Date:	5.12.63
No. Weeks In Chart:	24
Reached No. 1:	12.12.63
Total Sales:	1,750,000

The song that broke The Beatles in America and opened the floodgates for the so-called British invasion of the United States. Perhaps more than any other song, this tune represents Beatlemania.

Released in the UK one month before its cataclysmic arrival in the US, this song was The Beatles' first Christmas No. 1, replacing another of The Beatles' chart-topping classics, 'She Loves You'. The previous Christmas had seen *The Black and White Minstrel Show* top the album charts. This single's five weeks at No. 1 and the accompanying chart-topping album, *With The Beatles* – the first ever to sell over a million – changed everything.

This was the song that reinforced the home-grown 'Beatlemania' sparked off by 'She Loves You' (see No. 8), with one million UK sales in two days. The song's release was complemented by 'The Beatles Christmas Show', which involved the band appearing in a series of comedy sketches during an evening of light entertainment.

The song did for The Beatles in America what 'She Loves You' had done for them in the UK. It entered the US charts at No.1 and sold a million

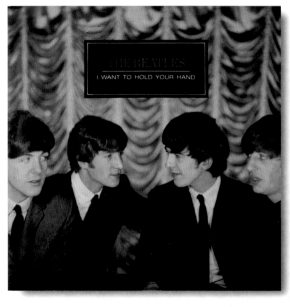

in three days. The commercial impact was so great that Prime Minister Douglas-Home called the besuited foursome 'my secret weapon'. The subsequent British invasion of the American charts was so complete that the federal government began denying visas to UK acts to stem the flood of British music stars outselling their US rivals.

After The Beatles had broken down the barriers, groups such as The Dave Clark Five, The Rolling Stones and The Searchers gleefully followed suit. Due to its global impact and subsequent cultural legacy (with worldwide sales in excess of fifteen million), this tune has been described by one rock critic as 'possibly the most important song in the history of rock'.

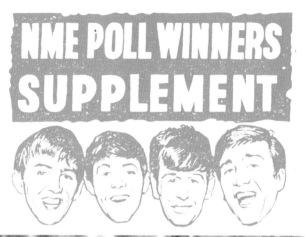

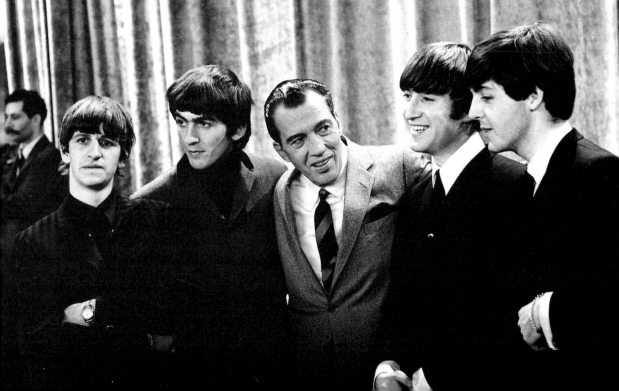

15 Barbie Girl
Aqua

Release Date: 25.10.97
No. Weeks In Chart: 26
Reached No. 1: 1.11.97
Total Sales: 1.722.418

The song received widespread criticism for being a lightweight novelty record; nonetheless, Aqua supporters pointed to the apparent sexual undertone of the lyrics.

Maybe not the purists' favourite, this release from the Danish Eurodisco act Aqua enjoyed remarkable chart success across the globe. Aqua was the musical offspring of Norwegian ex-TV hostess Lene Nystrøm, shaven-headed former DJ Rene Dif, and friends and former petrol station work colleagues Claus Norreen and Soren Rasted.

A previous collaboration between Claus and Soren on one of Denmark's most popular children's films had primed them for future fame. 'Barbie Girl' was the third single from the quartet and their first international success. At home in Denmark, their previous records had sold 250,000 copies, representing one in twelve households in that country.

Those figures were soon dwarfed by 'Barbie Girl' statistics, including more UK sales than The Beatles' 'Can't Buy Me Love' and 'Imagine' by John Lennon, and four million sales worldwide. Legal wrangles with the Barbie doll manufacturer Mattel were successfully negotiated (Japanese girl band Shonen Knife had previously name-checked the doll with

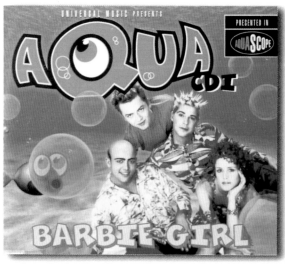

their rather less poppy 'Twist Barbie') and the debut album *Aquarium* went on to sell an unbelievable 14 million copies worldwide. Combined singles and album sales for Aqua are approaching 30 million. Another chart-topping success came with the excellent lead song from the soundtrack to the film *Sliding Doors*, namely 'Turn Back Time'.

'The musical offspring of Norwegian ex-TV hostess Lene Nystrøm, shaven-headed former DJ Rene Dif, and friends and former petrol station work colleagues Claus Norreen and Soren Rasted.'

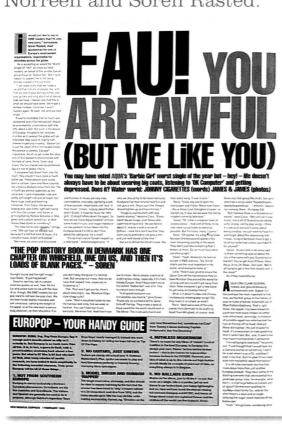

EAU! YOU ARE AWFUL
(BUT WE LiKE YOU)

You may have voted AQUA's 'Barbie Girl' worst single of the year but – hey! – life doesn't always have to be about wearing big coats, listening to 'OK Computer' and getting depressed. Does it? Water world: JOHNNY CIGARETTES (words) JAMES & JAMES (photos)

"THE POP HISTORY BOOK IN DENMARK HAS ONE CHAPTER ON WHIGFIELD, ONE ON US, AND THEN IT'S LOADS OF BLANK PAGES." — SOREN

EUROPOP – YOUR HANDY GUIDE

1. NOT FROM SOUTHERN EUROPE

2. NO GUITARS, JUST SYNTHS

3. MODEL, SINGER AND RUBBISH 'RAPPER'

4. RUTHLESS MODERNISM

5. NO BALLADS EVER

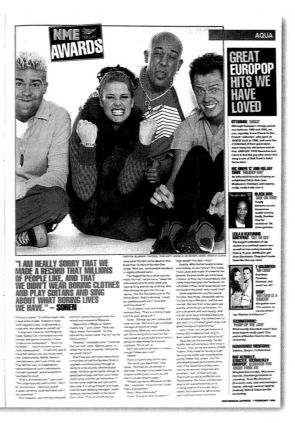

AQUA

GREAT EUROPOP HITS WE HAVE LOVED

OTTAWAN: 'D.I.S.C.O'

MC MIKER 'G' AND DEEJAY SVEN: 'HOLIDAY RAP'

BLACK BOX: 'RIDE ON TIME'

LEILA K FEATURING ROB'N'RAZ: 'GET THE GET'

2 UNLIMITED: 'NO LIMIT'

SNAP: 'RHYTHM IS A DANCER'

TECHNOTRONIC: 'PUMP UP THE JAM'

WHIGFIELD: 'SATURDAY NIGHT'

ACE OF BASE: 'ALL THAT SHE WANTS'

"I AM REALLY SORRY THAT WE MADE A RECORD THAT MILLIONS OF PEOPLE LIKE, AND THAT WE DIDN'T WEAR BORING CLOTHES AND PLAY GUITARS AND SING ABOUT WHAT BORING LIVES WE HAVE." — SOREN

16 Believe
Cher

Release Date: 31.10.98
No. Weeks In Chart: 28
Reached No. 1: 31.10.98
Total Sales: 1,672,108

This was not Cher's first foray into dance music – back in 1979, the disco-inflected 'Take Me Home' was a modest success, although she later confessed to hating it.

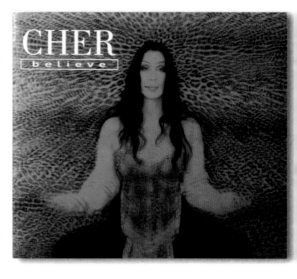

Cher is the biggest-selling female solo star in British chart history. Although this was seen as something of a 'comeback' single, Cher had in fact enjoyed three Top 20 hits (including the No. 1 charity single 'Love Can Build A Bridge') just over two years previously.

Cher has enjoyed her own prime-time TV show with Sonny Bono, international No. 1 hits, an Oscar-winning acting performance (for 1987's *Moonstruck*), yet has also fought against dyslexia, been pilloried by the anti-plastic surgery lobby, scoffed by critics for numerous album flops and even played in lounge bars to help fight off the IRS (Internal Revenue Service).

'Believe' gave her the best-selling single of her career, a transatlantic No.1 (for seven weeks in the UK – the year's best-seller) and secured the longest span between chart-toppers in US history – the hit came 24 years after 'I Got You Babe'. The song, a massive hit on the gay scene, later won an Ivor Novello songwriting award – a decision subjected to much derision from critics who scorned the simplistic lyrics. Nonetheless, the use of a vocoder on 53-year-old Cher's vocals has since proved highly influential. Her relationship with Sonny always shadowed her work, and when the latterday congressman was killed in a skiing accident in 1998, the world's media hounded Cher through Heathrow airport, despite the fact they had been separated for nearly 25 years.

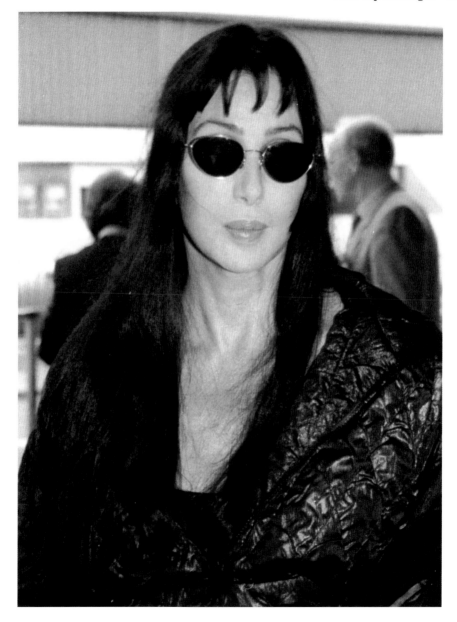

17

Perfect Day
Various Artists

Release Date: 29.11.97
No. Weeks In Chart: 21
Reached No. 1: 29.11.97
Total Sales: 1,548,538

The BBC had wanted to choose a song that would reflect the corporation's diverse range of musical tastes and broad cross-section of audiences. It was only natural, therefore, that the track should also draw in talent from a multitude of musical genres.

Belonging to that rare brand of single that has sold more than 1.5 million copies, this cover of a Lou Reed song was the centrepiece of the 1997 BBC 'Children In Need' charity fund-raising campaign.

The classic Reed ballad had originally appeared on his best-selling 1972 album *Transformer*. This beautiful re-working of the song was certainly musically accomplished – but perhaps even more impressive was the work that went on behind the scenes. The BBC managed to record, and also film for the accompanying video, a clutch of the world's greatest musical stars, including Bono, David Bowie, Lesley Garrett, Joan Armatrading, Elton John, Tammy Wynette and Tom Jones, as well as Lou Reed himself.

Each artist sang one line (Reed sang the first two and final lines), rather than using the hackneyed approach of potentially nauseating mass vocals – a fall-back of so many 'charidee' singles. This made the record a delightful production, and a tribute to the work of producers Mark Sayer Wade and Tolga Kashif, a.k.a. the Music Sculptors. The accompanying video was inter-cut with images of a garden, filmed at different moments – from sunrise to sunset – within the time frame of a single day, as the embodiment of almost everyone's notion of what constitutes a 'perfect day'.

The innovative nature of the project and the accompanying live event – embracing 6,000 concerts and 250 street festivals nationwide – helped make that year's 'Children In Need' one of the most successful ever.

According to the BBC, the single featured artists from the following genres: Britpop, blues, classical, country, easy listening, experimental, gospel, hip-hop, indie, jazz, opera, pop, rap, reggae, rock, soul, trip hop and world music.

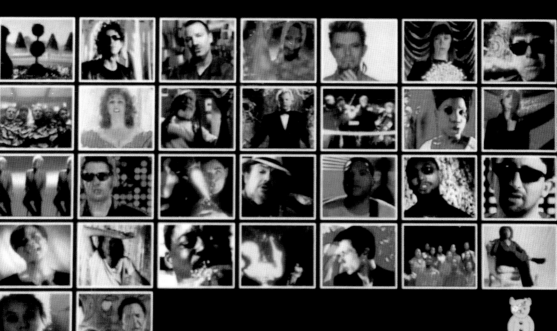

Perfect Day

BBC

ALL PROFITS TO BBC CHILDREN IN NEED

The '50s

Rock 'n' roll began in the '50s: so did the charts. What both needed to survive was a ready-made and hungry market – enter the teenager . . .

Up until the end of World War II, British adolescents were thought of either as children or as young adults, with no apparent period of transition between these two stages of life.

By the early '50s, however, changing economics and a growing awareness of a youth culture on the opposite side of the Atlantic were having a dramatic effect on this status quo. The new Labour government had ushered in an era of relative prosperity following the grim days of the wartime ration book. A national labour shortage meant that 15-year-old school leavers could secure well-paid jobs with reasonable ease. Suitably financed, these British youngsters were keen to consume – and rock 'n' roll provided them with the perfect commodity. Their anxiety to spend was fuelled by the dull certainty of eighteen months' military duty, as the prospect of National Service hung over their heads. The 'teenage consumer' was born, and society would never be the same again.

Rock 'n' roll had begun to blend the music of black culture, R&B and boogie with new – often white – performers, and its appeal was undeniable. It is said that Elvis spent every

TOMMY STEELE, MEL TORME, PAT BOONE
DICKIE VALENTINE, CYRIL STAPLETON—

News and articles in this issue

new MUSICAL EXPRESS

JOHNNIE SWAYS HIS WAY TO SUCCESS

PETULA IS 'FIRST LADY' OF THE HIT PARADE

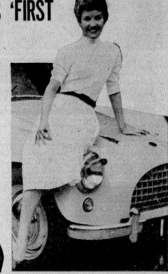

Petula Clark looks mighty happy—and why not? Her "With All My Heart" gained four places in the hit lists this week. She n o w occupies Number Eleven spot and is the only female singer in the first 18 places. Well done, Pet !

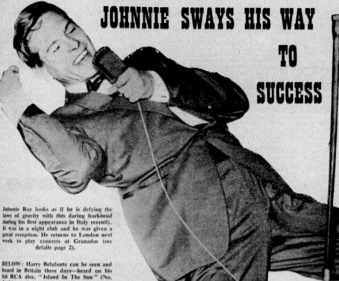

Johnnie Ray looks as if he is defying the laws of gravity with this daring backbend during his first appearance in Italy recently. It was in a night club and he was given a great reception. He returns to London next week to play concerts at Granadas (see details page 2).

BELOW: Harry Belafonte can be seen and heard in Britain these days—heard on his hit RCA disc, " Island In The Sun " (No. 5 this week), and seen in the film of the same name.

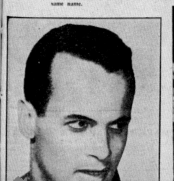

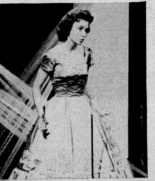

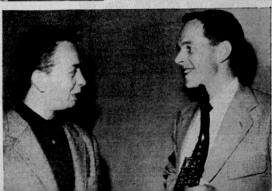

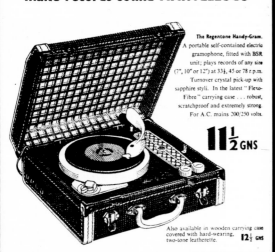
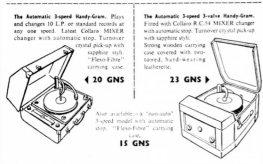
spare dime he could muster on buying records by African-American artists. Of course, with the new music came a new fashion. Prior to this fresh new import, 'youth style' had largely been a watered-down version of the parents' look. Now the battle lines were drawn. Influenced by images of early American rockers, the UK teenager craved the parental disapproval that rock 'n' roll provoked. The teddy boy of the '50s is seen as the first true teenage cult – albeit a predominantly working-class one.

The style drew as much from the fashions of the Edwardian period as it did from the rock 'n' rollers, pastiching as it did the upper-class dress in vogue in the early 1900s. The boys wore tight 'drainpipe' trousers, longer-than-usual jackets with trimmed collars and cuffs (called Drape coats, because of their cut), elaborate waistcoats, string ties and pointed-toe boots (called winkle-pickers) or crepe-soled suede shoes (called brothel creepers). They greased their hair back into elaborate quiffs. The girls wore the American-style full, circular, calf-length skirts, with their hair up – either in a 'beehive' or in a long ponytail sprouting from the crown. Teddy boys, teddy girls, or simply 'teds', had arrived.

General hysteria surrounding the teddy boys centred on late-night 'riots' at cinemas and similar acts of public disorder, and ensured that the phenomenon made front-page news. The film and television world was quick to spot the ratings winner that was the teenager. Performances on programmes such as *The Ed Sullivan Show* could often transform an artist into an overnight sensation. Likewise, cinema

NME MUSIC CHARTS

BEST SELLING POP RECORDS IN BRITAIN

Last	This		
1	1	MAN FROM LARAMIE	Jimmy Young (Decca)
2	2	BLUE STAR	Cyril Stapleton (Decca)
3	2	YELLOW ROSE OF TEXAS	Mitch Miller (Philips)
10	4	HERNANDO'S HIDEAWAY	Johnston Brothers (Decca)
5	5	ROSE MARIE	Slim Whitman (London)
6	6	COOL WATER	Frankie Laine (Philips)
8	7	ROCK AROUND THE CLOCK	Bill Haley Comets (Brunswick)
10	8	HEY, THERE	Rosemary Clooney (Philips)
4	9	EV'RYWHERE	David Whitfield (Decca)
9	10	HEY, THERE	Johnnie Ray (Philips)
12	11	HERNANDO'S HIDEAWAY	Johnnie Ray (Philips)
7	12	THE BREEZE AND I	Caterina Valente (Polydor)
15	13	I'LL COME WHEN YOU CALL	Ruby Murray (Columbia)
14	14	CLOSE THE DOOR	Stargazers (Decca)
13	15	LEARNIN' THE BLUES	Frank Sinatra (Capitol)
20	16	GO ON BY	Alma Cogan (HMV)
19	17	YELLOW ROSE OF TEXAS	Gary Miller (Nixa)
—	18	SONG OF THE DREAMER	Johnnie Ray (Philips)
17	19	I'LL NEVER STOP LOVING YOU	Doris Day (Philips)
—	20	BLUE STAR	Ron Goodwin (Parlophone)
—	20	MAN FROM LARAMIE	Al Martino (Capitol)

BEST SELLING SHEET MUSIC (BRITAIN)

Last	This		
1	1	BLUE STAR	(Chappells)
2	2	THE MAN FROM LARAMIE	(Chappells)
4	3	THE YELLOW ROSE OF TEXAS	(Maddox-Valando)
5	4	HEY THERE	(Frank) 2s.
3	5	EV'RYWHERE	(Bron)
6	6	HERNANDO'S HIDEAWAY	(Frank) 2s.
7	7	EVERMORE	(Rogers) 2s.
9	8	I'LL COME WHEN YOU CALL	(Michael Reine) 2s.
11	9	CLOSE THE DOOR	(Duchess) 2s.
8	10	EVERY DAY OF MY LIFE	(Robbins) 2s.
12	11	LEARNIN' THE BLUES	(C. & C.) 2s.
10	12	STARS SHINE IN YOUR EYES	(Peter Maurice) 2s.
13	13	UNCHAINED MELODY	(Frank) 2s.
15	14	LOVE ME OR LEAVE ME	(Keith Prowse) 2s.
19	15	GO ON BY	(Bluebird)
14	15	I WONDER	(Macmelodies) 2s.
17	17	COOL WATER	(Feldman) 2s.
18	18	SOFTLY SOFTLY	(Cavendish)
21	18	THE DAM BUSTERS MARCH	(Chappells) 2s. 6d.
16	20	JOHN AND JULIE	(Toff)
19	21	I'LL NEVER STOP LOVING YOU	(Robbins)
24	22	TWENTY TINY FINGERS	(F.D. & H.)
—	23	THE BANJO'S BACK IN TOWN	(Leeds) 2s.
23	24	HAVE YOU EVER BEEN LONELY	(L. Wright)

BEST SELLING POP RECORDS IN THE U.S.

Last	This		
2	1	Love Is A Many-Splendoured Thing	Four Aces
3	2	Autumn Leaves	R. Williams
1	3	Yellow Rose Of Texas	Mitch Miller
4	4	Moments To Remember	Four Lads
7	5	Shifting, Whispering Sands	Billy Vaughan
5	6	Ain't That A Shame	Pat Boone
8	7	Bible Tells Me So	Don Cornell
6	8	Tina Marie	Perry Como
13	9	Shifting, Whispering Sands	Rusty Draper
14	10	Only You	Platters
11	11	Yellow Rose Of Texas	Johnny Desmond
12	12	He	Al Hibbler
9	13	Black Denim Trousers	Cheers
10	14	Seventeen	Fontane Sisters
—	15	My Bonnie Lassie	Ames Brothers

BEST SELLING SHEET MUSIC (U.S.)

Last	This	
1	1	Autumn Leaves
2	2	Yellow Rose Of Texas
3	3	Bible Tells Me So
4	4	Love Is A Many-Splendoured Thing
5	5	Suddenly There's A Valley
8	6	He
9	7	Shifting, Whispering Sands
6	8	Wake The Town And Tell The People
10	9	Moments To Remember
7	9	Seventeen
13	11	Longest Walk
10	12	Ain't That A Shame
12	13	I'll Never Stop Loving You
—	14	My Bonnie Lassie
—	15	Love And Marriage

U.S. charts by courtesy of "Billboard."

box-office offerings pandered increasingly to the booming teen market. One of the most famous of all such films was the biker favourite, *The Wild One*, starring a youthful Marlon Brando. This black-and-white homage to the emerging biker scene was, effectively, a modern Western. Its story line drew on the much-publicised events of the 1947 Hollister bikers 'riot' for its backdrop. Brando, leader of the Black Rebels motorcycle gang, appears astride a gleaming black Triumph motorcycle wearing thigh-hugging denim jeans, bike boots, a tight-fitting zip-up black-leather bike jacket, and an almost paramilitary-style peaked cap tilted at a provocative slant.

Seen as overtly macho and even brutish at the time, it is notable that this iconic image has since been adopted – and to some extent subverted – by gay culture, attracted by its machismo. Further fuelling the 'forbidden' appeal of the film, *The Wild One* was not available for public consumption in the UK until some fifteen years after its 1953 US release – by which time it seemed dated and tame, as the 'moment' had passed. However, photographic images and stills from *The Wild One* had landed in Britain via the press years before its UK release.

The '50s also saw numerous other crazes, such as trad jazz (see No. 58) and skiffle. Yet it was rock 'n' roll that stayed the course. Bill Haley was at its core, despite his age and appearance (see No. 31), while England's answer to Elvis came in the form of an energetic 17-year-old by the name of Cliff Richard (see No.'s 68, 90).

18

(Everything I Do) I Do It For You
Bryan Adams

Release Date: 29.06.91
No. Weeks In Chart: 25
Reached No. 1: 13.07.91
Total Sales: 1,527,824

Adams would class himself primarily as a songwriter – his 45 million album sales complement writing credits for Bachman-Turner Overdrive, Ian Lloyd and Prism.

This was the lead single from the movie *Robin Hood: Prince of Thieves* starring Kevin Costner, a $400-million-grossing box-office smash that sent sales of the track through the stratosphere. The song's sixteen weeks at UK No. 1 smashed the 36-year record for the most consecutive weeks at the top (beating Slim Whitman's twelve weeks with 'Rose Marie'). This transatlantic chart-topper also became the first million-seller in the UK since Jennifer Rush's 'The Power Of Love' six years previously (see No. 37).

This success was in startling contrast to the prevailing commercial trend at the time. The year 1991 saw more singles chart than ever before, as records joined the listings at a higher slot, but for briefer periods – making Adams' achievement all the more remarkable.

Having broken into the UK psyche with the album *Reckless* in 1985, Adams reinforced his reputation with a slew of cleverly honed yet simple rock tunes, promoted with an exhaustive live schedule that at one point saw him play 283 gigs in the same year. This song was co-written

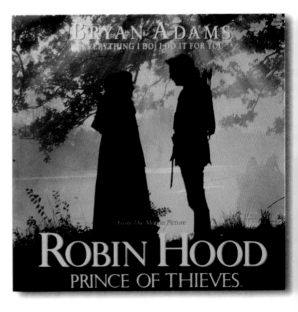

by Adams with Michael Kamen and Mutt Lange (super-producer/future husband of Shania Twain), based around a melody Kamen had been keeping since the '60s. The ten million sales pipped Whitney Houston's 'I Will Always Love

You' to the post as the most successful commercial single ever released until 1997 (see No.'s 1 and 36). The song was critically lambasted in the UK, but in the US gave Adams a Grammy and an Oscar nomination. In 1992, a cease and desist order was served on a former Ku Klux Klan member using the tune to soundtrack his campaign for political office.

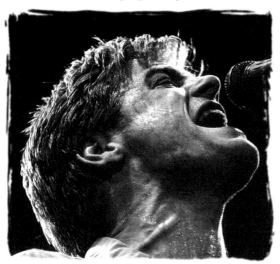

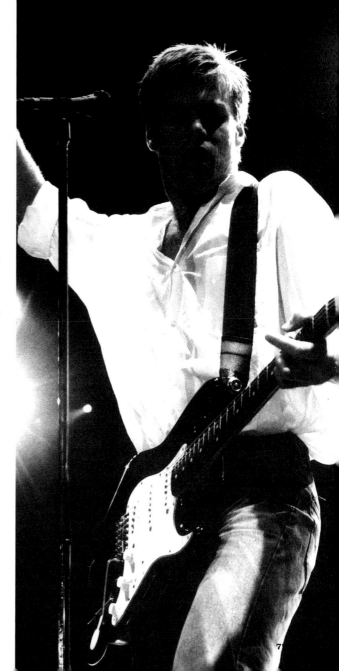

19

Tears
Ken Dodd OBE

Release Date:	2.09.65
No. Weeks In Chart:	24
Reached No. 1:	30.09.65
Total Sales:	1,521,000

Dodd can boast singles in his back catalogue that have outsold George Michael, Whitney Houston, John Lennon and even Elvis' most impressive efforts.

Although Liverpudlian Dodd is renowned for his oddball personas, famous tickling-stick and comedic incarnations such as 'Professor Yaffle Chuckabutty, Operatic Tenor and Sausage Knotter', he is also a hugely successful recording artist.

A veteran of the seaside summer seasons of the '50s, Dodd's church-choir background and the trend in the '60s for comedians to close their stand-up routines with a song, pushed the perennially popular entertainer towards a chart career. 'Tears' was a remake of a 1929 Rudy Vallee song – its follow-up single, 'The River', earned Dodd two songs in the Top Ten at the same time. The million-and-a-half-selling 'Tears' was usurped only by The Rolling Stones' 'Get Off Of My Cloud'; 1965 was the year the Stones and Bob Dylan were huge, The Beatles played Shea Stadium in the US as Beatlemania exploded and The Who were unsettling the music press everywhere, a context which makes Dodd's achievements all the more remarkable. In his mid-30s at the time, the salesman-turned-comedian racked up eight Top 20 hits in total – this single was 1965's best-seller, ahead of 'We Can Work It Out/Day Tripper'. Oddly, his two comic songs of that year, 'Where's Me Shirt?' and 'Song of the Diddymen', were relatively unsuccessful.

'The King of Comedy' has also fronted TV series, defeated the taxman in court, played Malvolio in Shakespeare's *Twelfth Night* and is one of the biggest box-office stars in the theatre.

KEN DODD

A British counterpart of all those sweet-corn discs the Americans have been churning out lately can be found in **Ken Dodd's** "Tears" (Columbia).

Ken solos with humming support in some passages, then is joined by the sing-along group in the chorus—all set to an easy-going soothing lilt.

Romantic ballad of the type in which **Ken** specialises, "You And I" was written by **Norman Newell** and **Michael Carr.** Has a very colourful backing.

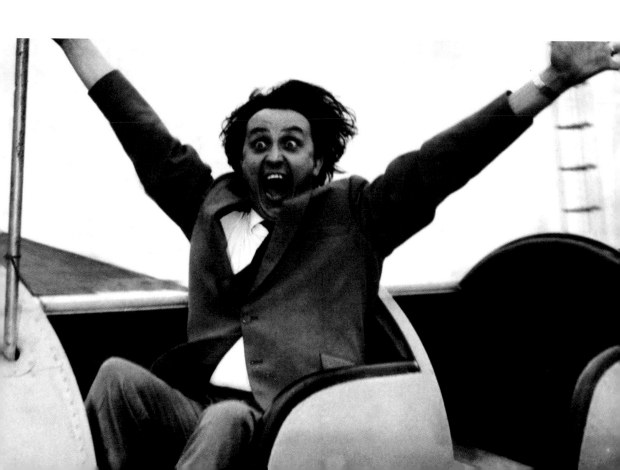

20 Can't Buy Me Love
The Beatles

Release Date: 26.03.64
No. Weeks In Chart: 17
Reached No. 1: 2.04.64
Total Sales: 1,520,000

The single was taken from the hugely successful film and album project, *A Hard Day's Night*, which sold one million copies in America inside four days.

This single coincided with Beatlemania travelling across the Atlantic. At the start of this year the US-christened 'Mop Tops' were unknown in the US, but by the month of this song's release (March) they could account for 60 per cent of all record sales in that country (although it was actually 'I Want To Hold Your Hand' that 'broke' America – see No. 14).

Record advance orders in the UK were matched by two million of the same in America. When this song hit No. 1 Stateside, The Beatles could boast an unprecedented complete sweep of the Top Five plus three of the top four albums. The song also enjoyed massive international success, with No. 1 status in scores of other countries across the globe.

Written and sung by McCartney, this is the band's third biggest-selling single (see No.'s 8 and 14). It was taken from the album of their first feature film, which

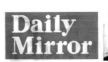
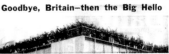
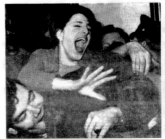
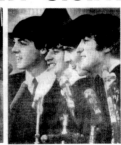

was completed in between constant touring and US success – the double Oscar-nominated *A Hard Day's Night*. The album of the same name contained, for the first time, no covers and is seen by some as the finest of the early period Beatles. This single also marked the band's first performance on *Top of the Pops* and was covered by Ella Fitzgerald only one month after

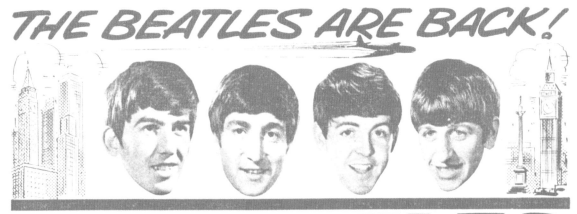

THE BEATLES ARE BACK!

THE BEATLES
Can't buy me love PARLOPHONE R 5114

the original. It set a then UK record by selling over 1.2 million singles in one week – some achievement for a tune that was actually an afterthought during a French recording session. Providing some food for thought, Beatles' archivists claim that the harmonies which were removed from the final version would have made the song even better.

21 Summer Nights
John Travolta and Olivia Newton-John

Release Date: 16.09.78
No. Weeks In Chart: 19
Reached No. 1: 30.09.78
Total Sales: 1,515,000

Grease remains a firm favourite for nostalgists, students, karaoke bars and parties the world over. The single is one of two songs in this list to come from the soundtrack.

The second single in the list from the *Grease* soundtrack (see also No. 6), this was also a No. 1 hit for the Travolta/Newton-John partnership. Enjoying seven weeks at the top slot, the single was joined by 'Sandy' at No. 2 and, remarkably, ' Hopelessly Devoted To You' at No. 4. *Grease* went on to gross $340 million at the box office, making it the most successful musical film of all time.

Oddly, the phenomenon proved alarmingly quick to fade away. Only a year after dominating the world's charts, Travolta released an album containing a compilation of his hits from both *Saturday Night Fever* and *Grease*, which barely scraped into the US Top 200.

Olivia Newton-John enjoyed a further UK No. 1 with ELO on the track 'Xanadu', from the critically mauled film of the same name, and a ten-week stint on top of the US charts with 'Physical'.

Since *Grease*, she has released ten albums, won scores of awards, been awarded an OBE by the Queen and, in 1992, engaged in a successful battle against breast cancer.

Travolta endured a career slump in the '80s, only to return to form as an ultra-cool actor in watershed movies such as *Pulp Fiction*. The double Oscar-winning actor has since become one of Hollywood's biggest-grossing stars ever. In 2002, Travolta bought his own Jumbo jet for $60 million – when told that only one private runway in America would fit a Jumbo, he bought that, too.

Of course, the '50s look and greaser appeal of the movie was never as enduring or as symbolic as Travolta's three-piece, white flared suit and medallion in the '70s disco feature *Saturday Night Fever*. Nonetheless, the appeal of *Grease* does not seem to diminish. A musical revival in London's West End and a 1998 twentieth anniversary re-issue have only added to the film and soundtrack's iconic status.

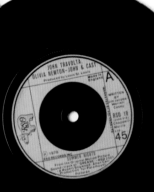

**JOHN TRAVOLTA AND
OLIVIA NEWTON-JOHN:
Summer Nights (RSO).
CHRIS BLAKE AND
HONEY BROWN: Summer
Nights (Weekend).**   Despite
the fact that neither John is
remotely human, they have
been given superior flash
dance pop material that no one
could fail with. Because their
faces fit. They are the best
combination of their type since
Anne Nightingale and Alan
Black, which proves two
tediums do make a something.

"You're The One That I
Want" was delightful. This,
with its careful local and period
colloquial realism and
unrepresentative bounce and
colour, is passable, with the
bass player again deserving
most of the royalties.

Chris Blake and Honey
Brown are two British TV
comedy actors who perform an
exact copy of the original. For
reason's sake, why?

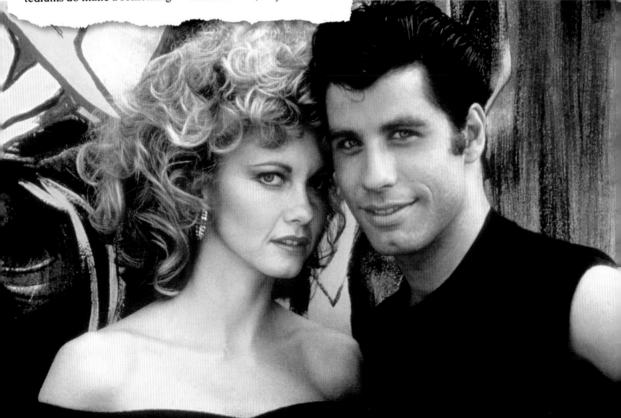

22 Two Tribes
Frankie Goes To Hollywood

Release Date: 16.06.84
No. Weeks In Chart: 21
Reached No. 1: 16.06.84
Total Sales: 1,510,000

The apocalyptic sound of 'Two Tribes', set against a backdrop of continuing Cold War tensions, managed perfectly to capture the zeitgeist of the time.

After the cataclysmic impact of Frankie Goes To Hollywood's debut single, 'Relax' (see No. 7), many observers doubted they could repeat either the commercial success or indeed the musical brilliance of that awesome opener. Incredibly, with the follow-up 'Two Tribes', the Liverpool five-piece actually managed to go one better artistically.

Composed on the same night as 'Relax' and in the same disused police cell rehearsal room, 'Two Tribes' gave Frankie a duo of historically important singles. This time, their self-proclaimed 'protest song' stayed at No. 1 for nine weeks and in turn dragged 'Relax' back up to No. 2, buoyed by full Radio One backing second time around.

This double chart-topping domination was a feat shared only by The Beatles and a solo John Lennon. The superb Godley and Crème-produced video offered up sweaty footage of Reagan and his Russian counterpart Chernenko lookalikes grappling in a wrestling ring. This was supplemented by a chilling voiceover by actor Patrick Allen, whose sinister Orwellian tones advised citizens on the dangers of nuclear fallout and the safest ways to dispose of dead relatives while avoiding radiation (a script taken from genuine government papers). This truly frightening morbidity found several new leases of life in the various multiple remixes – on both seven and twelve inch, not to mention picture-disc formats – that Frankie would make their speciality.

Their later debut double-long player, *Welcome To The Pleasure Dome*, was a multi-platinum smash, and their third single, 'Power of Love', also hit the top spot (making them at that point the only act other than Gerry and the Pacemakers to enjoy three No. 1s with their first three singles).

However, Frankie never really improved on this spate of opening classic tracks. Their 'temporary' split, first announced in spring 1987, eventually became permanent, leaving Johnson to fight record company ZTT successfully in the courts over his contract – a decision seen as a pivotal shift in the balance of power in the music industry.

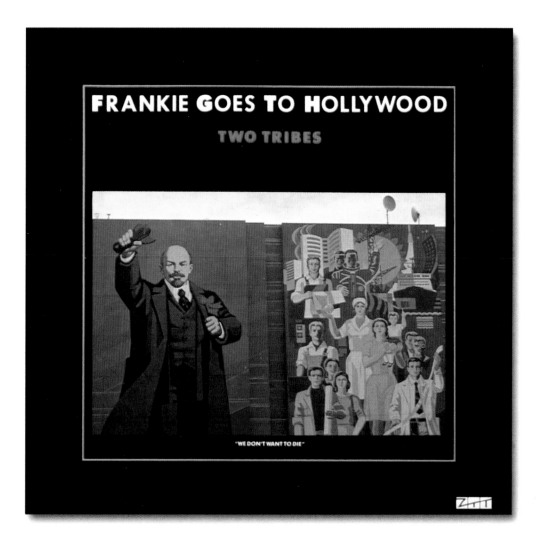

23 Imagine
John Lennon

Release Date: 1.11.75
No. Weeks In Chart: 42
Reached No. 1: 10.01.81
Total Sales: 1,486,581

Lennon's most famous solo record hit the No. 1 spot almost ten years after its initial 1971 release as a track on the transatlantic No. 1 album of the same name.

The eventual 1975 single release of 'Imagine' came some four years after the appearance of the album of the same name, and only after consistent radio play had championed the tune. The song reached No. 6, which at that point was only Lennon's fourth-best effort. He admitted later that he wished he had jointly credited Yoko Ono for the Utopian classic, which he said drew heavily on her paperback book *Grapefruit*. At the time, the song's pseudo-religious musings offended many groups, but it is now seen as an anthem of peace and the very antithesis of the violence which ended his life.

Lennon had just come out of a five-year self-imposed retirement as a house husband when he was shot dead outside his New York apartment in December 1980 by obsessed fan Mark Chapman (for whom he had earlier signed his new album). In the immediate aftermath, Lennon's record sales rocketed, with this single being the first of three tracks to climb to the No. 1 spot within eight weeks of his death.

Conspiracy theorists whispering about the establishment's dislike for the ex-Beatle did little to dampen the public's enthusiasm for Lennon, giving him three of the Top Four singles in January 1981. A movie of home video footage and unreleased songs, also entitled *Imagine*, was released in 1988 and saw a re-issued version of this single reach No. 45.

Stupendous B-side of the Century

JOHN LENNON: Imagine (Apple) This is the oldie referred to, and the B-side is "Working Class Hero". Like "Imagine", which presumably needs no description from me, "Hero" has never appeared on a single before, chiefly because it contains That Word — twice — and so is unlikely to get airplay.

Or was. We shall see.

Like a lot of Lennon's solo work, both songs are impressive, and they are very impressive *despite* rather than *because* of the personal philosophy they presumably express(ed).

Even in 1970, the cracks were beginning to show; naivety and confusion raising their heads. I mean, *imagine* all the people, living for today — not a very inspiring thought; and lines like "you think you're so clever and classless and free", and "first you must learn to smile as you kill" are/were dead giveaways: Lennon, after all, isn't/wasn't a *working class* hero (though he's a hero all right) and is/was basing his ideas here on secondhand experiences.

It doesn't/didn't matter; his sincerity, his personality, are/were large enough to get him by.

DAILY Mirror

Wednesday, December 10, 1980   12p

JOHN LENNON
shot dead
in New York
Dec 8 1980
DEATH
OF A
HERO

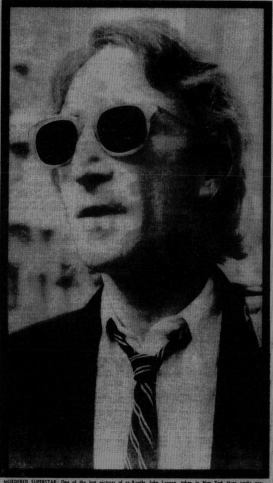

MURDERED SUPERSTAR: One of the last pictures of ex-Beatle John Lennon, taken in New York three weeks ago.

24 Baby One More Time
Britney Spears

Release Date: 27.02.99
No. Weeks In Chart: 22
Reached No. 1: 27.02.99
Total Sales: 1,450,154

This globally huge debut single was a perfect slice of tightly composed modern pop, fizzing with infectious vocals and world-class production.

From among the legions of post-Spice Girls wannabes, one saccharine pop star emerged triumphant – Britney Spears. However, it was the accompanying video, shot at California's Venice High School (the same one as in the 1978 movie *Grease* – see No. 6) that caused furore and moral outrage.

In the video, a then under 16-year-old Britney and assorted school chums, all dressed in skimpy, 'Catholic-school-girl' pleated skirts, with their white school blouses tied up to reveal inches of underage flesh, cavorted and danced their way around the hallways and gymnasium. It was somewhat more engaging than the original storyboard idea, which had been a rather dull 'Britney Power Ranger'.

The moral majority cried foul, accusing Spears' lyrics of inciting misogynistic violence, but their complaints helped lift Ms Spears and her wholesome Louisiana persona to the top of the charts. This was just the first of many colossal-selling records for the prodigious Britney, a fact that made her record company, Jive – home also to Backstreet Boys and N*Sync

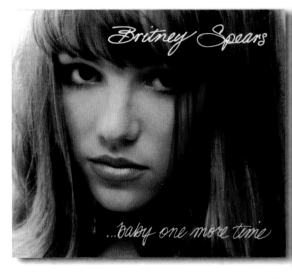

– one of the most successful labels in the world. Nearly 1.5 million UK sales tell just one aspect of the phenomenon – this track alone went on to top global sales of nine million copies.

It is worth noting that cover versions by Travis and Barenaked Ladies have not sold quite as heavily.

'The moral majority cried foul, accusing Spears' lyrics of inciting misogynistic violence, but their complaints helped lift Ms Spears and her wholesome Louisiana persona to the top of the charts.'

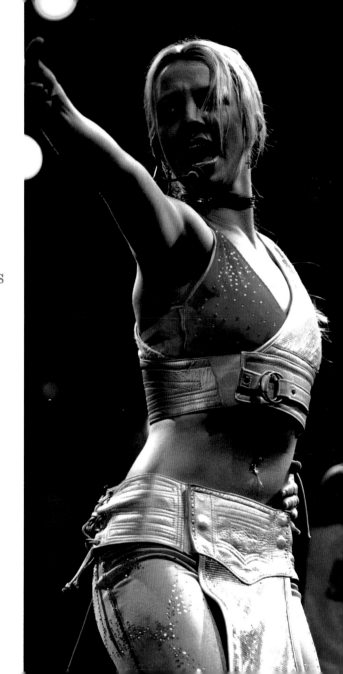

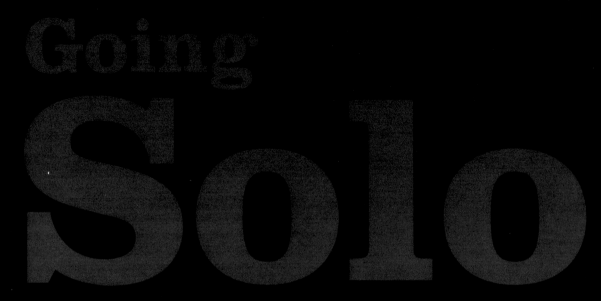

Going Solo

The Winners and Losers

'Should I stay or should I go?' The song's refrain may surface when a band hits troubled times, but does taking care of 'number one' necessarily bring a slew of No. 1s?

One thing is abundantly clear from the list of big names in this book: not one of the artists responsible for these Top 100 songs has achieved bigger sales as a solo star with a single than with a group.

George Michael is the list's biggest solo winner. 'Careless Whisper' was his debut solo release and fell only 50,000 short of Wham!'s best single, 'Last Christmas'. However, this may have been facilitated by the fact that Michael released the saxophone ballad while Wham! were still an active group.

He has since gone on to surpass the sales of this '80s pop duo, bolstered by huge success in America – although his 2002 single 'Shoot The Dog', which some saw as critical of the US, saw him berated by a nation still smarting from the terrorist atrocities of 11 September 2001.

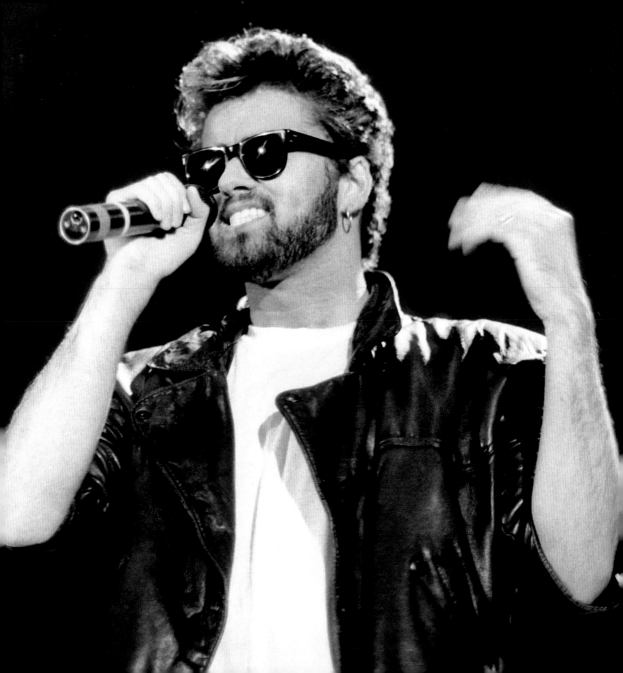

who could not be expected to take second place to subsequent solo careers – the critical plaudits tended at first towards George Harrison and John Lennon, while it was McCartney's new group, Wings, which enjoyed the highest post-Fab Four single success (see No. 4). Pink Floyd also experienced varying degrees of success, although the open-air spectaculars of Roger Waters were not matched by hefty singles success (see No. 78).

Other big names on the list have enjoyed a solo success that seems minuscule compared to the individual's breath-taking achievements within a band. Queen's May, Mercury and Taylor all dabbled with solo records or new band line-ups; Holly Johnson of Frankie Goes To Hollywood collected just two Top Five hits on his own. All Saints splintered into three, with the Appleton sisters forming a self-titled duo, leaving Melanie Blatt and Shaznay Lewis to go their solo ways. Similarly, Steps fragmented into three new careers after their acrimonious split in late 2001, with H & Claire earning most of the immediate media attention.

When the Spice Girls were on top of every chart in the world, few could have guessed that their latter-day solo careers could prove so fleeting. The band that brought Girl Power to the world then gave us a reincarnated Ginger Spice, in turn replaced by a yoga-mad, UN Goodwill Ambassador Geri. But commercial hits were never matched by critical acceptance. Emma Bunton, in the wake of her initial success with the No. 1 'What Took You So Long', quickly faded, as did Scary Spice Mel B

much-publicised battle for the top slot against Groovejet Featuring Sophie Ellis Bextor, Posh Spice Victoria Beckham's solo career also stuttered. Despite Sporty Mel C enjoying sound album success and a Top Three chart single with the late Lisa Left Eye Lopes of TLC, the Spice Girls' all-conquering girl-band prowess was a quantum leap away from the sporadic solo success of the respective members.

Often the weight of critical acclaim attached to a band seems to suffocate even credible attempts to break out a new career. New Order, who themselves worked major miracles by successfully crawling out from under the critical spectre of Joy Division, never enjoyed lengthy solo success.

Frontman Barney Sumner formed Electronic with ex-Smiths guitar maestro Johnny Marr, long-armed bassist Peter Hook formed the excellent, albeit short-lived, Monaco, leaving the self-effacing Stephen Morris and Gillian Gilbert to form the muted The Other Two. Likewise, Kevin Rowland of Dexy's Midnight Runners enjoyed sporadic acknowledgements from the critics until the lambasting he received for his comeback solo project in 1998, which saw some of the music industry's most venomous critical pillorying ever.

Solo careers have never been predictable. Boyzone's lead singer Ronan Keating was perhaps an obvious bet for chart success as a solo star. Yet while he enjoyed a platinum debut solo album and a best-selling autobiography, his former band mate Stephen Gately pierced the Top Ten only once with 'New Beginning

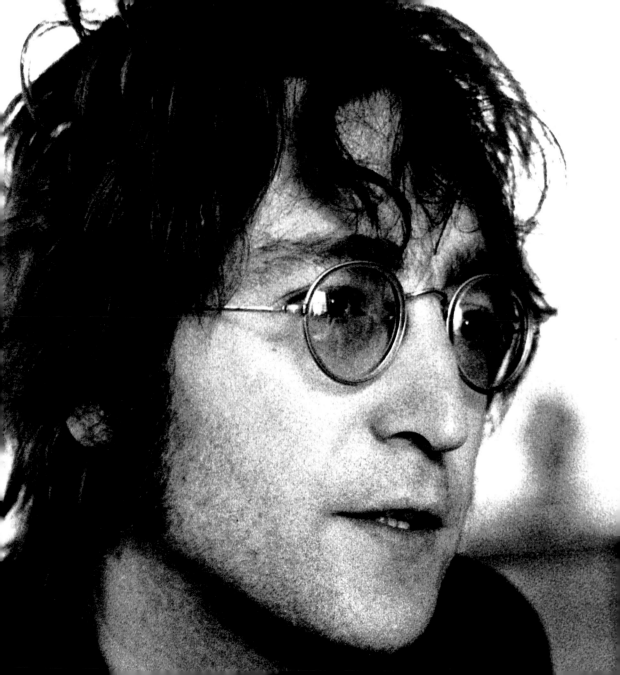

Mikey Graham only hit the Top 20 once, while Keith Duffy found new expression acting on top TV soap *Coronation Street*.

Take That, like Boyzone, provided distinct winners and losers in the solo race, even if these roles were very much against the predicted form. A few pundits placed their money on the teen-girl favourite Mark Owen, but his brief foray into solo stardom provided only two Top Five hits, including the curious Lennon pseudo-parody of 'Child'. Hot favourite to become 'the next George Michael' was Take That's chief songwriter, Gary Barlow.

With accomplished ballads such as 'Back For Good' and pop classics like 'Pray' already in his repertoire, Barlow seemed a sure-fire winner. Not so. His solo career began well, with two chart-toppers ('Forever Love' and 'Love Won't Wait'), but thereafter his chart success slipped.

Barlow's difficulty in fulfilling his apparent legacy was made all the more remarkable by the phoenix-like emergence of Robbie Williams as the new millennium's favourite entertainer. Despite public battles with various vices, Robbie's multi-platinum albums, singles and huge sell-out tours have shaped him as perhaps the most versatile performer of the current generation – yet 'Angels', the ballad which turned around a rapidly fading solo career, could not make this list.

Like Keith Duffy from Boyzone, Culture Club's Boy George eventually found an alternative career, this time around in DJ-ing. After a tempestuous career post-Culture Club, which included a debut No.1 solo single ('Everything I Own') followed by four singles that made it into

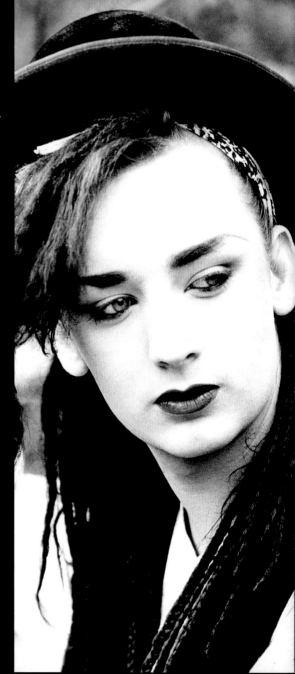

that did not, Boy George became one of the most highly sought-after – and best-paid – club DJs in the world (see No. 29).

Olivia Newton-John was already a chart solo star when she released 'You're The One That I Want' (see No. 6), even having her own greatest hits album, yet her short-lived partnership with Travolta in 1978 brought in much heavier sales; Rod Stewart genuinely broke free of The Faces to establish himself as one of the great solo rock stars of the modern era. Blondie's Debbie Harry never competed with the pure pop-punk quality or the chart success of the band she fronted; Adam Ant hit the top after the Ants but then, in an abrupt change of direction, headed off to Los Angeles to pursue an acting career.

One of the few groups for whom solo careers has meant great success for all the members are the Fugees. After the global smash album *The Score* and the breakthrough single 'Killing Me Softly' (see No. 41), all three members of the group – Wyclef Jean, Pras and Lauryn Hill – enjoyed critical acclaim and heavyweight commercial success.

Wyclef became the producer of choice to numerous superstars, as well as having hits with bands as diverse as Queen, Destiny's Child and U2 lead singer Bono and, latterly, producing tracks for Tom Jones. Pras released 'Ghetto Superstar' to huge sales. But it was Lauryn Hill who made the greatest impact after the group's demise. She scooped a bagful of Grammies and millions of album sales with her impressive solo debut album *The Miseducation of Lauryn Hill,* which entered the *Billboard* charts at No. 1.

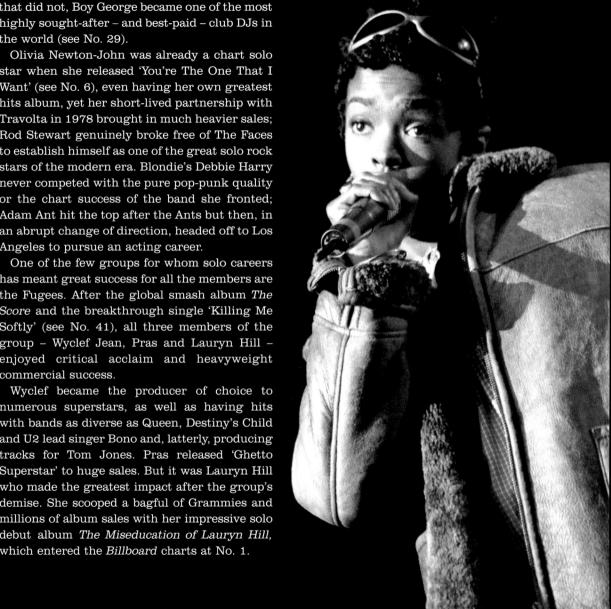

25 Don't You Want Me?
Human League

Release Date: 5.12.81
No. Weeks In Chart: 16
Reached No. 1: 12.12.81
Total Sales: 1,430,000

This was the first truly commercial meld between previously avant-garde electro-music and pop – a watershed moment in the history of electronic music.

The lop-sided haircut of former hospital porter, frontman and co-writer Phil Oakey provided Human League with an unmistakable image. Named after a computer game, Human League achieved only modest chart success initially, but their pivotal moment came when they started working with the brilliant maverick producer Martin Rushent.

Within months, they were atop the charts with this, their fourth Rushent collaboration. The superb video perfectly captured the song's sentiments as the two protagonists verbally jousted with one another over a failed relationship. This song was the first platinum single since 'Mull of Kintyre' (see No. 4) and gave Virgin Records their first ever No. 1 single.

The corresponding masterpiece and No. 1 album, *Dare!*, was a five-million-seller globally and Virgin's second best-seller ever, behind Mike Oldfield's instrumental classic, *Tubular Bells*. Six months after its UK chart success, this song topped the US charts, helping to open the door to a host of British bands in America, including Duran Duran and Spandau Ballet.

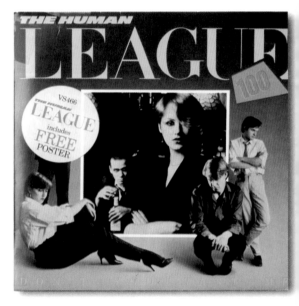

Although their sound quickly dated, they did enjoy another US No. 1 with the Jimmy Jam and Terry Lewis-produced 'Human' in 1986. Human League are now regarded as one of the seminal bands in electronic music history.

The Human League give away a poster that shows half a dozen Norman Hunters in mean mood. We mutilated our copy and shoved it under the Kitty Litter. It is proving very waterproof, being glossy. Samson Oakey — who resembles Phil McNeill at the height of punk — needs to have a haircut and the stuffing knocked out of him. But it takes two to do it (duet) wrong. This could be a swinging little song if given to two black singers with GREAT VOICES. Phil and moll sound sallow and callow. So many people should be silent songwriters. You could be in folklore instead of on *Top Of The Pops*. Look at Phil Spector. No, don't look at him like that!

The Human League must stop using the singles chart as an agony column sometimes. And my scout tells me there *are* no cocktail bars in Sheffield. And they're too sensitive. They could learn a lot from. . .

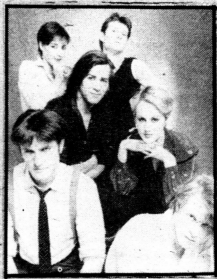

LEAGUE GO PLATINUM

THE HUMAN LEAGUE single 'Don't You Want Me' is being claimed by Virgin as the first platinum selling record in this country for four years — they say that, according to their statisticians, it hasn't happened since Paul McCartney's 1977 Christmas hit 'Mull of Kintyre'. Well, that's their theory, and anyone who disagrees should contact Virgin — not *NME!* One point which can't be argued is that the album from which it came, 'Dare', is now Virgin's biggest selling LP since their very first — 'Tubular Bells' by Mike Oldfield — having sold over 750,000 copies, and well on the way to a million.

26 Last Christmas/Everything She Wants
Wham!

Release Date: 15.12.84
No. Weeks In Chart: 24
Reached No. 1: N/A
Total Sales: 1,420,000

One of the classic pop Yuletide hits from one of the finest pop acts of the '80s – yet the song never made it to No. 1.

Released after George Michael had already launched a parallel solo career (see No. 34), this was Wham!'s seventh Top 20 hit – but the song was kept one place short of the top slot by the might of Bob Geldof's Band Aid single, 'Do They Know It's Christmas?' (see No. 2), on which Michael also sang. As with that track, this effort by Wham! is a perennial festive favourite, boosting its total close to the 1.5 million mark.

After first being turned down by all the major record labels they approached, Wham! enjoyed a rapid rise to fame, blossoming from complete unknowns to three hit singles in under two years. George Michael's cohort in the swoonsome twosome ('Teen Dreams come true' was how one *NME* article dubbed the pair) was his old school friend Andrew Ridgeley. Ridgeley maintained that Wham! were purely tongue-in-cheek. The critics weren't so convinced – and the fans didn't care.

A ground-breaking show in Peking, China, masterminded by pop maestro manager Simon Napier-Bell, ensured that Wham! made a notable contribution to music history, over and above their already impressive commercial

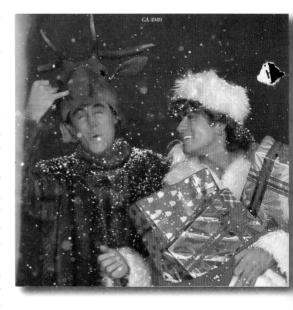

success. They were also the first Western pop group to have a single released behind the red curtain. The farewell gig at Wembley stadium attracted 80,000 screaming fans – and Michael and Elton John duetted on 'Candle in the Wind 97' (see No. 1). 'Last Christmas' remains the biggest-selling record never to hit No. 1.

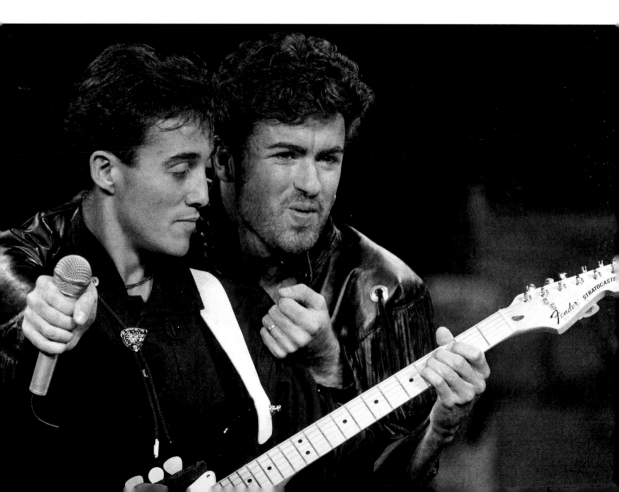

27 I Feel Fine
The Beatles

Release Date: 3.12.64
No. Weeks In Chart: 14
Reached No. 1: 10.12.64
Total Sales: 1,410,000

> The opening rasp of guitar feedback was claimed repeatedly by John Lennon to be the first time that this had been deliberately recorded for a commercial release.

Knocking The Rolling Stones' 'Little Red Rooster' off the top slot, this track was The Beatles' second consecutive Christmas No. 1 – following the previous year's festive smash, 'I Want To Hold Your Hand' – and a song of which Lennon was particularly proud.

The key bluesy riff that runs throughout the song revealed Lennon's love of R&B and his pride in it was never to diminish. When he played at Madison Square Garden with Elton John in 1975 – in what was to be Lennon's last major concert appearance – he was overheard playing the 'I Feel Fine' guitar riff as he strolled on to the stage.

This single rounded off a monumentally successful year for The Beatles – a year that at one stage had seen them boast 30 (yes, 30) songs in the US singles charts. Incredibly, at one point during 1964 they held all five top positions in the *Billboard* Hot 100, a feat that no one has come even close to equalling since. In the UK, this single stayed at the top for five weeks, and was complemented in the album charts by the year's best-seller, *Beatles For Sale*.

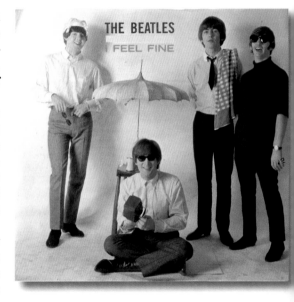

The Fab Four's tangential success and acclaim was also blossoming – Lennon had recently won a literary prize for his nonsensical book *In His Own Write*, his acceptance speech for which was, 'Thank you very much. You've gotta lucky face.'

TEN TOP CHART CERTS (STARTING
WITH THE BEATLES, OF COURSE)

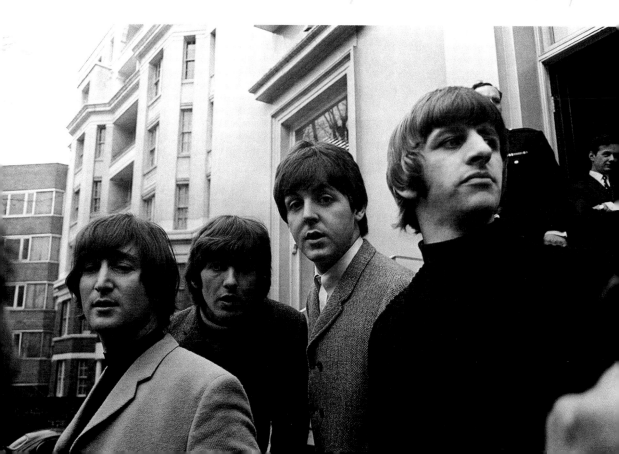

28 I'll Be Missing You
Puff Daddy and Faith Evans

Release Date: 28.06.97
No. Weeks In Chart: 21
Reached No. 1: 28.06.97
Total Sales: 1.409.688

This single was the biggest hit to date for Bad Boy Entertainment, formed after Puffy's meteoric rise to pre-eminence within the hip-hop record industry.

When revered East Coast rapper Notorious B.I.G. was shot dead in March 1997, his best friend and record label owner Sean Combs, a.k.a. Puff Daddy, released this tribute. Based around a sample of The Police's classic 'Every Breath You Take', the song features B.I.G.'s wife Faith Evans on vocals alongside Puffy. This No. 1 entry into the charts was the biggest hit to date for Puffy's Bad Boy record label and enjoyed much UK radio play after the death of Princess Diana.

A Harlem-born paperboy turned A&R executive at Uptown Records, Puffy shot up through the ranks of the music biz – initially, he made his name by dancing, promoting hip-hop concerts and producing acts such as Father MC, Mary J Blige, and Jodeci. Bad Boy was run at first from his own apartment, then later aligned to Arista (who were rumoured to have paid $75 million to help set up Bad Boy Entertainment).

A feud with Tupac Shakur and Suge Knight of West Coast's Death Row Records dissipated when Tupac was murdered and Knight imprisoned. The death six months later of B.I.G.

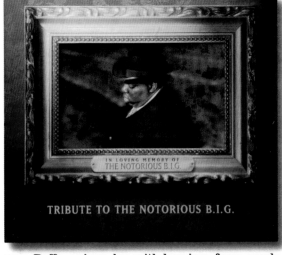

TRIBUTE TO THE NOTORIOUS B.I.G.

saw Puffy grieve by withdrawing from work altogether for months, before returning first with 'Can't Nobody Hold Me Down' and then this pop-infected slice of mainstream hip-hop (both taken from the solo album No Way Out). Criticised by many for his over-reliance on samples, and for commercialising the sound of the underground, Puffy (or P Diddy as he now likes to be known) has since set up his own designer label, established a children's charity, been acquitted on a gun-related charge and had a high-profile affair with actress/singer Jennifer Lopez. Combs calls himself 'an entertainer', not a rapper.

Oasis bumped by Puff Daddy

OASIS were knocked from the top of the singles charts at the weekend after Puff Daddy's 'I'll Be Missing You' reclaimed the Number One slot.

Some industry insiders had predicted that the Oasis record would be Number One for as long as a month, but despite becoming the fastest-selling single this year in its first week of release, sales dropped off in the second week. The Puff Daddy Notorious BIG tribute single meanwhile had sold more than 700,000 copies by the end of last week. Sting, whose 'Every Breath You Take' is sampled on the single, is reported to have made £400,000 in royalties.

Before Oasis were toppled from the Number One slot, the band marked their success with an appearance on *Top Of The Pops* last Friday – during which the audience invaded the stage.

A spokeswoman for the show said that it was only the second time on the programme's history that a spontaneous stage invasion had happened – the first time was in November 1991 while Nirvana performed 'Smells Like Teen Spirit'.

The show's producer Chris Cowey was undaunted by the fact that Oasis chose to mime on the show, which has recently revamped its format to encourage live performances.

"We encourage bands to play live and sing, but it's up to them," he said.

29 Karma Chameleon
Culture Club

Release Date: 17.09.83
No. Weeks In Chart: 20
Reached No. 1: 24.09.83
Total Sales: 1,405,000

Androgynous styling and quips such as 'preferring tea to sex' made Boy George one of *the* faces of the '80s.

The second and final No. 1 of their highly controversial career, after 1982's 'Do You Really Want To Hurt Me?', this was the biggest-selling UK single of 1983. Fuelled by the growing power of MTV, the harmonica spliced melody, George's soulful voice and unique image, this was Culture Club's only US No. 1 – highlighting an unexpected American fascination with his blurring of sexual roles.

Emerging from the decadence of the nightclub scene of the early '80s, the outrageous cross-dressing style of former hairdresser's model Boy George (George O'Dowd) belied his roots in suburban Kent. After a brief stint in Malcolm McLaren's Bow Wow Wow, Bowie fanatic George hooked up with veteran punk drummer Jon Moss and Culture Club was born. It was the turn of pop, not rock, to shock.

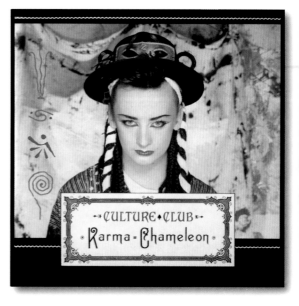

This single was part of the so-called 'second invasion of the US' which saw acts such as Human League (see No. 25) and Dexy's Midnight Runners (see No. 48), along with Culture Club, fill up one-third of the *Billboard* charts. The corresponding album, *Colour By Numbers*, was also a US smash, only beaten by Michael Jackson's epochal *Thriller*. After this peak, the band's career faded away almost as quickly as it had arrived. A solo George later enjoyed a No. 1 with a version of the David Gates/Bread tune 'Everything I Own'. A period of stasis and a role within the Hare Krishna movement pre-empted a return to favour, which saw George emerge as one of the most sought-after DJs in the world.

SINGLE OF THE WEEK

CULTURE CLUB: Karma Chameleon *(Virgin)* Karma: quite literally, any act that appears in consecutive singles columns with the same author. Chameleon: a thin sneaky lizard that absorbs its current background and grins a lot (though slap one on a piece of kilt and they cry like babies). And Culture Club chameleoze the West Coast. Lying long in the sun they become as the sound of the surf. It's 'Marakesh Express' and Todd Rundgren and The Eagles and the opening beats of 'You're So Good To Me' by Beach Boys. It's peace and love, team; perky, free and easy, clever and crafty and this country's very next number one hit single. I love it pretty much to pieces and seem to play it all the time. Ha! So it wasn't a mystical man-dress after all George. You've been wearing a kaftan, you silk-voiced foul mouthed old she-wolf.

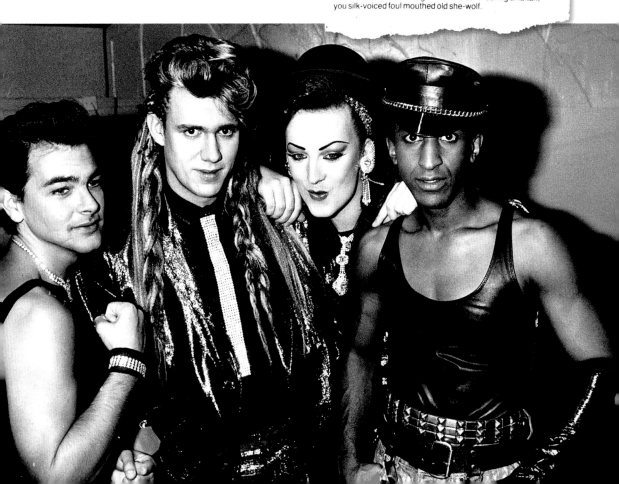

30 The Carnival Is Over
The Seekers

Release Date: 28.10.65
No. Weeks In Chart: 17
Reached No. 1: 25.11.65
Total Sales: 1,400,000

Australia's first UK chart-topping act and a beacon of mellowness in the midst of Beatlemania.

This was the second No. 1 success of the year for Australian vocal group The Seekers, after 'I'll Never Find Another You' – a track written for them by Tom Springfield, who wrote five of the group's Top Ten hits. The single found itself sandwiched between 'Get Off Of My Cloud' by The Rolling Stones, which it replaced at No.1, and The Beatles' classic double A-side 'Daytripper/We Can Work It Out', which in turn bumped The Seekers off the top slot after three weeks.

Leading man Keith Potger was born in Colombo, in what was then Ceylon (now Sri Lanka), in 1941. The only non-Australian of the group, he had nevertheless lived in Melbourne all his life. He was in the Escorts, which mutated into The Seekers in the early '60s. The Seekers' soft tones and gentle harmonies proved extremely popular with the record-buying public, despite being rather at odds with the musical approach of many of the beat groups. After this brace of chart toppers, success was a little more muted, aside from the famous 'Georgy Girl' and 'Morningtown Ride', before the band split up in 1968.

Following this, Potger went on to form the New Seekers (see No. 81). Incidentally, their version of Paul Simon's 'Some Day, One Day' gave Simon his first UK hit.

" THE CARNIVAL IS OVER "/" WE SHALL NOT BE MOVED" (Columbia). CONSIDERABLY slower than their last two hits, but again written by Tom Springfield, Judith opens solo with just tambourine and rhythm—then the boys enter with unobtrusive humming, and eventually they break into unison with lush strings to add depth.

It's a very attractive and plaintive ballad, beautifully harmonised, with an insistent beat. Builds strongly. FORECAST : The fans will have to readjust themselves to the Seekers after such a long absence, but I'm sure this is Top Ten material. FLIP : Again it's Judy to the fore in this traditional gospel number, which steadily works its way up to a vibrant hand-clapping climax.

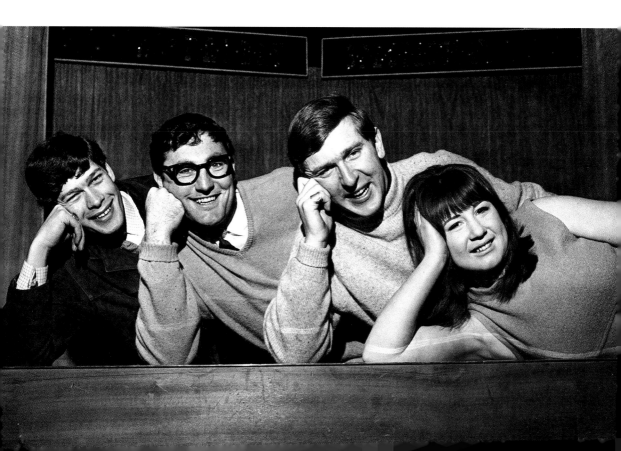

31 (We're Gonna) Rock Around The Clock
Bill Haley and His Comets

Release Date: 7.01.55
No. Weeks In Chart: 57
Reached No. 1: 25.11.55
Total Sales: 1,392,000

This song is the very foundation block of rock 'n' roll – performed, ironically, by a 30-year-old Haley and co-written by Max Freedman, a songwriter in his sixties.

Haley, a former country and western singer and sometime yodeller, was the improbable torch-bearer for the incendiary new art of rock and roll. Abandoning the Stetson-clad efforts to ape Hank Williams which characterised his routine during the late '40s, Bill Haley re-invented this cover version of a little-known Sunny Dae track with seminal results.

The record's initial release achieved only a modest No. 17 in the charts (Haley only recorded the live staple as a favour to his manager), but eleven months later the record shot to No. 1 after being used under the opening credits of the Glenn Ford film, *The Blackboard Jungle*, a story of juvenile delinquency in a New York High School.

Five further re-entries in the charts (a unique feat) sent sales of the earliest entry in this book soaring past the million mark. Not bad for a song which Decca Records had listed initially in their catalogue as 'a foxtrot'.

Haley can probably boast more rock 'n' roll 'firsts' than any other artist: the first rock 'n' roll chart hit, 'Rocket 88', a cover of the R&B smash; his first sessions at Decca producing this, the first rock 'n' roll No. 1; the first rock 'n' roll riots; the first artist to introduce the form to white America; and, with his kiss curl and raucous live set, Haley was the first rock 'n' roll icon (albeit an unlikely one).

This song was the very first UK million-seller, a watershed moment and the signal that rock 'n' roll was an entirely fresh genre, rather than merely a youth fad. Blind in his left eye, overweight and 30 years old when this song hit the big time, Haley nonetheless opened the floodgates for every rock 'n' roll singer after him.

Unfortunately, his roles in various movies, including *Rock Around The Clock*, seemed only to highlight his age and image in stark contrast to the youthful sexuality of Elvis and others. Even so, when this 'anti-establishment' film was first screened, cinemas across the UK reported

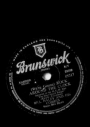

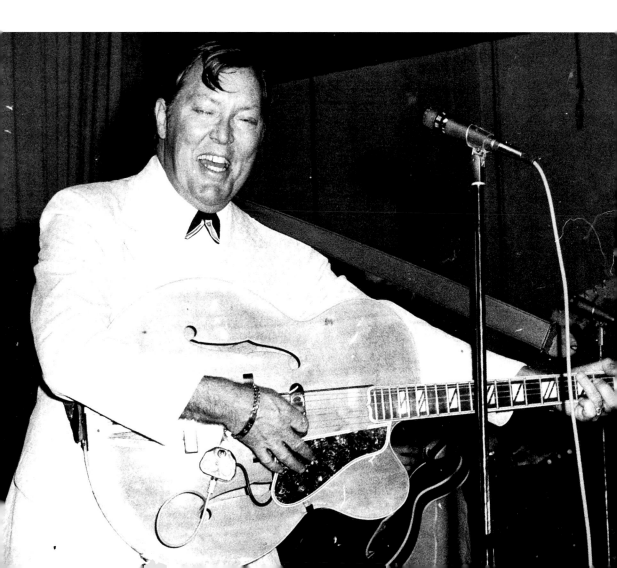

seats being torn up and widespread rioting, fuelled by the establishment-baiting teddy boys, most famously at London's Trocadero (mirroring similar riots across the US).

After the success of his glory years (a relatively short period, after all, between 1955 and 1956), Haley drank heavily and is said to have lived out his final days riddled with paranoia, in his garage whose walls he had painted black. On his death in 1981, his neighbours were reported to be unaware of his phenomenal musical past.

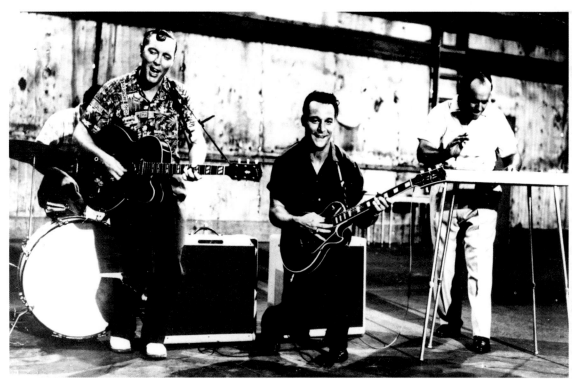

There's plenty of room for all tastes— so please don't 'knock the rock !'

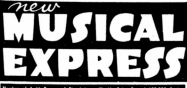

No. 578   EVERY FRIDAY PRICE 6d.   February 1, 1957
Member of Audit Bureau of Circulation : Weekly Sales Exceed 100,000 Copies

'Rock 'n' Roll Personality Parade'
—See page 6

Bill Haley writes in this issue

February 'Hit Parade' on sale this week-end

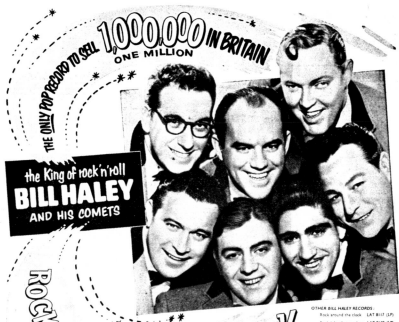

THE ONLY POP RECORD TO SELL 1,000,000 IN BRITAIN
ONE MILLION

the King of rock'n'roll
BILL HALEY
AND HIS COMETS

ROCK AROUND THE CLOCK

05317

AMERICAN RECORDINGS
Brunswick
RECORDS

OTHER BILL HALEY RECORDS :
Rock around the clock   LAT 8117 (LP)
Rock 'n' roll stage show   LAT 8139 (LP)
also OE 9278-80 (EPs)

TWO BRAND NEW 78/45s FROM THE
FILM " *DON'T KNOCK THE ROCK* "

Don't knock the rock   05640
Hook, line and sinker   05641

Shake, rattle and roll   05338
Two hound dogs Razzle dazzle 05453
See you later, alligator   05530
The Saints rock 'n' roll   05565
Rockin' through the rye   u5582
R.p.it up   05615

BRUNSWICK LTD. Branch of THE DECCA RECORD COMPANY LTD
1-3 BRIXTON ROAD, LONDON, S.W.9

32 We Can Work It Out/Daytripper
The Beatles

Release Date: 9.12.65
No. Weeks In Chart: 12
Reached No. 1: 16.12.65
Total Sales: 1,385,000

This festive hit capped a remarkable year for The Beatles, which at one point saw them enjoy no fewer than three albums in the Top Ten album charts.

This double A-side was The Beatles' third consecutive Christmas No. 1 (for five weeks), bumping The Seekers' 'The Carnival Is Over' from the top spot, although the latter eventually sold 1,500 more copies (see No. 30). In parts, the record showcased a heavier-than-usual rock sound from the Fab Four.

Publicly, John Lennon preferred the rockier 'Daytripper', complete with one of music's most instantly recognised guitar riffs, to the cleaner pop sound of 'We Can Work It Out', which was said to be a blend of two previously unfinished songs. 'Daytripper' was Lennon's jibe at so-called part-time or 'weekend hippies'; McCartney sang lead vocals as he could accommodate the high notes in each verse more easily. The flip side of the record was a perfect blend of the McCartney/Lennon dual muse. This release earned The Beatles their fifth Gold disc and their ninth No. 1.

The single came in the same year as the Fab Four received their MBEs, smoked marijuana at Buckingham Palace and provoked dozens of former soldiers to return their own award medals in disgust. This was also the second year that Beatlemania had possessed America. The legendary Shea Stadium show in front of 55,000 hysterical fans was pop music's biggest-grossing concert in history.

Back at home, The Beatles also played their last gig at the Cavern Club – the gloomy basement near Liverpool's docks which had first made them famous – for which they were paid the sum of £3,000.

Unbeknown to their millions of fans, the release of this single coincided with what would turn out to be The Beatles last-ever full UK tour. Four months later, John Lennon made his (somewhat) controversial 'We're more famous than Jesus' comment.

Following this single, The Beatles delved into more experimental musical projects, hints of which had come with the No. 1 *Rubber Soul* album of this same mid-'60s period.

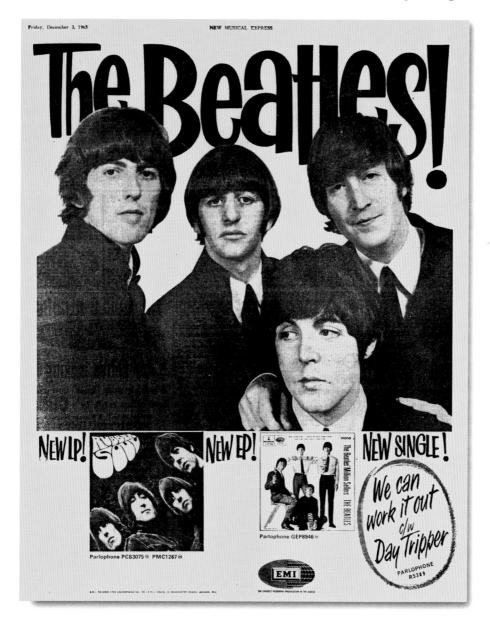

33 YMCA
Village People

Release Date: 25.11.78
No. Weeks In Chart: 26
Reached No. 1: 6.01.79
Total Sales: 1.380.000

The fancy dress attire of New York's gay underbelly provided the image, while a sextet of singing actors supplied the vocals for what was to be the first of three huge hit singles for this exuberant ensemble.

Looking back now at the flagrantly homosexual stereotypes that were the Village People – the Indian, the construction worker, the policeman, the G.I., the cowboy and the biker – it is hard to believe that much of mainstream society did not cotton on to the group's gay inspiration.

Conceived by French-born New York producer Jacques Morali, 'YMCA' was the first of three million-selling hit singles for this shamelessly camp act, although only this single passed the seven-figure mark in the UK alone (benefiting from the record-breaking market for single sales at that time).

In the early days, the gay underground championed the group, but later – when disco reached its fevered peak – the gay scene grew tired of them. A conservative and sexually repressed UK, however, took the single one place higher than its No. 2 success in America.

Amazingly, even after the release of 'Macho Man' and the strident 'I Am What I Am', there were still some members of the record-buying public who remained blissfully oblivious to the band's roots.

The group's fortunes plummeted after their ill-fated film *Can't Stop the Music*, but they have since re-emerged – enjoying renewed success year after year as perennial party favourites.

However, the irony of thousands of aunts and uncles cheerfully singing this thinly veiled paean to youthful gay sex is usually completely lost on the countless wedding receptions it has graced since its release. And this, despite the inclusion of innuendo-loaded lines such as 'It's fun to stay at the Y-M-C-A', they have everything for you men to enjoy, you can hang out with all the boys'.

The Village People mastermind, Morali, lost his life in 1991 due to Aids-related illness.

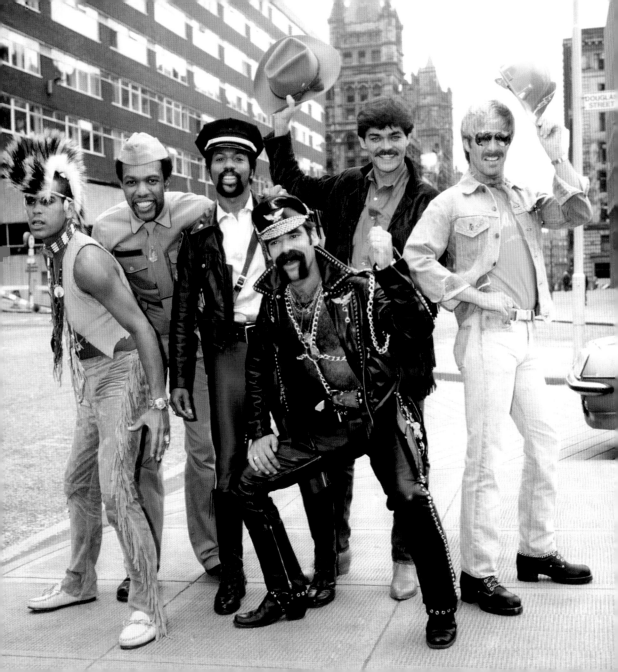

34 Careless Whisper
George Michael

Release Date: 4.08.84
No. Weeks In Chart: 17
Reached No. 1: 18.08.84
Total Sales: 1,365,995

'Careless Whisper' is something of a career oddity – written three years before it was released; released three years before the accompanying solo album.

George Michael is that rare thing in pop – a bona fide teen sensation who has successfully morphed into a serious singer/songwriter, with equal levels of commercial success. As one half of the coiffured, pearly-white pop duo of Wham!, alongside former school buddy Andrew Ridgeley, Michael sold 38 million records in only four years – showing them to be the perfect group for the designer '80s.

Yet only three months after Wham!'s own first chart-topper, 'Wake Me Up Before You Go Go', Michael released his debut solo track, a song included in his first-ever publishing deal. Even back in 1982 when Wham! were first breaking through, he'd mentioned a potential solo single he'd written at the age of eighteen (purportedly on a bus), describing it as a 'soul ballad'.

The stylish sophistication of 'Careless Whisper' laid the perfect foundations for Michael's acclaimed latterday songwriting reputation. The No. 1 hit was dedicated to his parents and won him an Ivor Novello award. In America, it was released conversely as 'Wham!

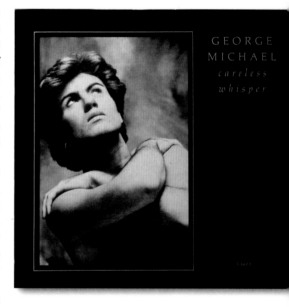

GEORGE MICHAEL *careless whisper*

Featuring George Michael' and also sold a million copies on its way to the top slot. A second solo track, 'A Different Corner', was also released before Wham! finally split in 1985. Michael subsequently became the first white

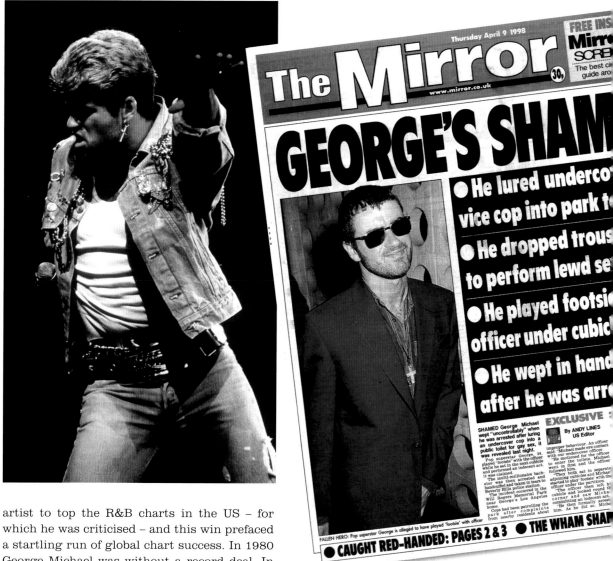

Thursday April 9 1998

The Mirror

www.mirror.co.uk   30p

FREE INS
Mirror
SCRE
The best ci
guide aro

GEORGE'S SHAM

- He lured underco
  vice cop into park t

- He dropped trous
  to perform lewd se

- He played footsi
  officer under cubic

- He wept in hand
  after he was arr

EXCLUSIVE

By ANDY LINES
US Editor

SHAMED George Michael wept "uncontrollably" when he was arrested after luring an undercover cop into a public toilet for gay sex, it was revealed last night.

Pop superstar George played "footsie" with the officer while he sat in the next cubicle and performed an indecent act, it was claimed.

The multi-millionaire bachelor was them arrested and handcuffed and taken in tears to Beverly Hills police station.

The incident occurred in the Will Rogers Memorial Park near George's Los Angeles home.

Cops had been patrolling the park after complaints from nearby residents about

improper behaviour. An officer said "Michael made eye contact with our undercover officer.

"He motioned for the officer to enter the toilets. Michael went in first and the officer followed him.

"They both sat in separate adjoining cubicles and Michael started to play 'footsie' with the officer under the partition.

"The officer then left the cubicle and looked round the corner and saw Michael committing an indecent act.

"He then formally arrested him. As he did so, Michae

FALLEN HERO: Pop superstar George is alleged to have played 'footsie' with officer

● **CAUGHT RED-HANDED: PAGES 2 & 3** ● **THE WHAM SHAM**

artist to top the R&B charts in the US – for which he was criticised – and this win prefaced a startling run of global chart success. In 1980 George Michael was without a record deal. In 1990 he was reputed to be worth £65 million.

35 Release Me
Engelbert Humperdinck

Release Date: 26.01.67
No. Weeks In Chart: 56
Reached No. 1: 2.03.67
Total Sales: 1,365,000

Although enjoying popularity at the same time as The Beatles, Humperdinck had more in common with 'master crooners' such as Frank Sinatra, Tony Bennett and Dean Martin than with the Fab Four.

Born in 1936 into a military family of twelve based in Madras, India, as plain Arnold George Dorsey, Engelbert Humperdinck has since become one of the world's greatest balladeers. After the family moved back to England and settled in Leicester, Dorsey learned his trade by doing the rounds of the clubs and pubs of the East Midlands, initially as a sax player.

Humperdinck's stage name in those early days was Gerry Dorsey, because of the impeccable Jerry Lee Lewis impression he performed. Engelbert still does impersonations to this day, and has included Elvis Presley along with his big rival, Julio Iglesias, in his mimicry.

Notably, his humorous stage shows belie his extreme vocal power and impressive three-and-a-half octave range. Originally a career in engineering had awaited Humperdinck, but this had to be postponed while he served his two years of National Service. On being demobbed, a six-month attack of tuberculosis threatened to ruin his budding musical career.

Fortunately, everything changed in 1966 when he returned with a name change and his former room-mate Gordon Mills as manager. He found his odd-sounding new monicker in a musical dictionary, naming himself after the nineteenth-century classical German opera composer behind Hänsel and Gretel.

At early shows, he was supported by Jimi Hendrix and, deliberately avoiding his fans to preserve his mysterious image, would often exit venues via a bathroom window. This song, his version of the country classic 'Release Me', was his debut smash and the biggest seller of 1967. In the late '90s, Engelbert released a dance version of this, his most commercially successful single (see also No. 52).

The amazing recovery of ENGELBERT HUMPERDINCK

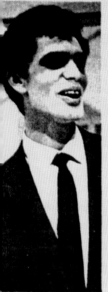

THEN as GERRY DORSEY in [19]61, Engelbert on "Thank Your Lucky Stars", nominated as star of the future by Adam Faith. But he was—as he looks—ill.

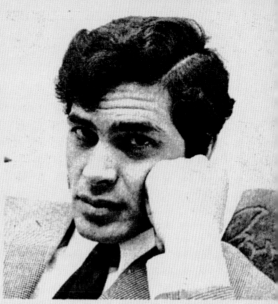

AND NOW as ENGELBERT HUMPERDINCK fully recovered from illness and worry, now a big star after a great struggle, he relaxes for the photographer.

THIS week let us all raise our glasses and drink to the health of Engelbert Humperdinck, who tops the NME Chart with "Release Me." I am, for one, delighted that he's made it big at last. Not only because of his sheer talent and perseverence, but because he made it against almost impossible odds.

By NORRIE DRUMMOND

Engelbert—or Gerry Dorsey as he was then—began his recording career [in] 1958 when Decca issued his first disc "Mr. Music Man". The record flopped and Gerry and Decca parted company but he continued making a reasonable living as a singer.

During the next three years he slowly built up a reasonable reputation through [TV] appearances on shows such as ["Oh] Boy." People started recognising him in the street and he was always being asked for his autograph.

Steady work

He had made several more records [for] different companies and work was pretty steady—in fact the future seemed very promising indeed.

"I always had the feeling that before my illness I had achieved a slight amount of success and I at least wanted to regain that."

He started recording again but still he had no success and meanwhile other singers were racing past him up the chart.

"I can't say I wasn't upset getting nowhere while other people were making it," he admitted.

Then early last year came the [...]

turned from Belgium when I met him and was enthusing over the audiences there.

"They're unbelievable. Everywhere we played was absolutely packed to capacity and the boys are wilder than the girls."

Engelbert Humperdinck has succeeded in what he set out to do—to get to No. 1.

"I don't care if I never get another hit record. I've achieved my ambition and now I'm happy."

Personally, I think it's just the beginning for Engelbert.

WHO'S WHERE

36 I Will Always Love You
Whitney Houston

Release Date: 14.11.92
No. Weeks In Chart: 29
Reached No. 1: 5.12.92
Total Sales: 1,355,055

This staggering blockbuster of a single saw sales across the world rocket to in excess of 8.6 million.

Houston had already racked up over 50 million album sales when this song became her biggest hit to date. The hit, a cover of Dolly Parton's 1982 song, was taken from the soundtrack to *The Bodyguard*, in which she gave an acclaimed debut acting performance opposite Oscar-winning actor-director Kevin Costner. The original screenplay was written years before, reputedly with Steve McQueen and Diana Ross in mind. The on-screen chemistry between Costner and Houston helped the film gross over $400 million.

The former model and backing singer for Chaka Khan broke through in 1985, with the ballad (her forte) 'Saving All My Love For You' making her an instant rival for the previously all-conquering Madonna. The daughter of a gospel singer and cousin of Dionne Warwick, Houston's reported five-octave vocal range is matched only by a select few (future rival Mariah Carey, for instance).

This song represented a critical return to form after the muted response to her third album *I'm Your Baby Tonight*. It enjoyed ten weeks at UK No.1, making it that year's best-seller. The soundtrack sold over 33 million

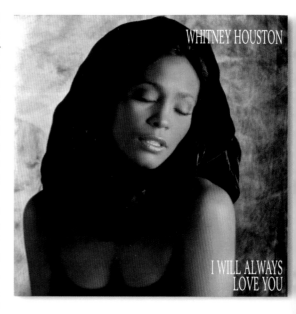

copies (one million in the first week in the US), at the time a world record.

Shortly after *The Bodyguard*, Houston gave birth to a baby girl, fathered by husband and singer Bobby Brown. Her recent career has been plagued by bouts of ill health and tabloid rumours of drug problems.

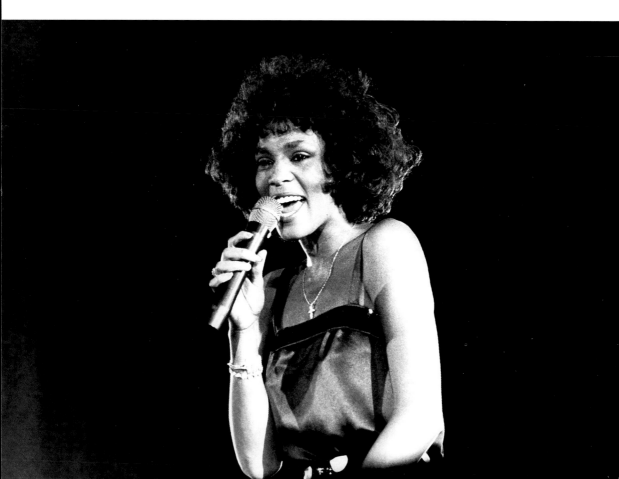

The '60s

The deaths in January 1959 of Buddy Holly, Richie Valens and Big Bopper in a plane crash near Clear Lake, Iowa, USA, left the music world reeling – and effectively brought to an end the first phase of rock 'n' roll.

The first generation had lost so many stars that a substantial 'power vacuum' was left. At first, the US-derived influences remained, with 'The Twist' and smartly dressed skiffle bands enjoying huge popularity. With both Cliff and Elvis apparently eschewing rock 'n' roll, music and youth culture seemed somewhat listless – but not for long.

No band has been written about as widely, nor cited as influences to such an extent, nor indeed achieved so much as The Beatles (see No.'s 8, 14, 20, 27 and 32). The first half of the '60s was theirs, and with that world domination came the Merseybeat scene. Beatlemania not only spearheaded the first major invasion of the American charts by British acts, but also exported the accompanying style and culture across the globe. The availability of imported US records at Liverpool docks had played its part in the Merseybeat scene breaking in the first place. But now that the phenomenon was global, foreign admirers inevitably looked to

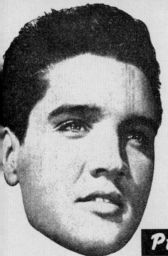

ELVIS
versus
CLIFF

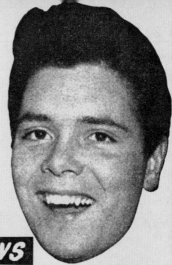

ELVIS PRESLEY and CLIFF RICHARD have, for the first time, discs released on the same day. Which one will win the chart race? The records are reviewed on page 4.

PERSONALITIES IN THE NEWS

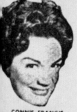

CONNIE FRANCIS
. . one-day London visitor and back in charts this week.

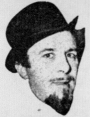

ACKER BILK
. . Gold Disc presentation for "Stranger On The Shore."

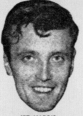

JET HARRIS
. . ex-Shadow, has first solo disc released this week.

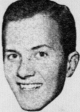

PAT BOONE
. . . presented a polished act as Palladium TV star.

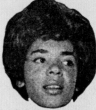

SHIRLEY BASSEY
. . . great Palladium variety debut on Monday.

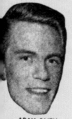

ADAM FAITH
. . entered charts again at No. 17 —as he likes it !

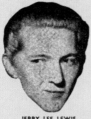

JERRY LEE LEWIS
. . . causing great excitement on his British tour.

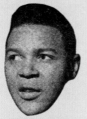

CHUBBY CHECKER
. . . continues to occupy two chart places with twist hits.

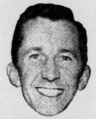

NORMAN VAUGHAN
. . . "swinging" out with first disc this week.

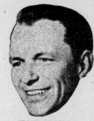

FRANK SINATRA
. . . eagerly awaited in London ; keeps twisting in charts !

London for inspiration. Suddenly, names like Carnaby Street and the King's Road were on the lips of people in cafés and bars all around the world: 'Swinging London' had arrived.

The product of tremendous media hype, 'Swinging London' was nonetheless the epicentre for musicians, photographers, models and cultural pioneers, including the anti-fashion waif and soon-to-be-supermodel Twiggy. Newspapers, television and radio all helped to publicise this burgeoning development so that, 'back home', provincial working-class teenagers started taking out 'lease' agreements to buy drums, cameras and guitars.

By 1963, everyone aspired to the neat suits, distinctive haircuts and lifestyle of the Fab Four. The Beatles had abandoned the greased quiffs of '50s rockers to don collarless jackets, Chelsea boots and the famous mop-top haircut.

It is ironic, perhaps, that a follicular style that did so much to help launch The Beatles (and the consequent global export of all things British) was actually the brainchild of a young German model, photographer and occasional hairdresser, Astrid Kirchherr. Astrid was the girlfriend of Stuart Sutcliffe, the so-called 'Fifth Beatle' who died of a brain tumour. Looking at the besuited Fab Four now, their haircuts seem to be the epitome of conservative style. Yet at the time, it was the first instance of men wearing their hair 'long' – the mop-top was even denounced from the pulpit as the precursor to the apocalypse.

While the '60s saw the fashion underground go overground, there was always a splinter group that stayed beneath the tabloid

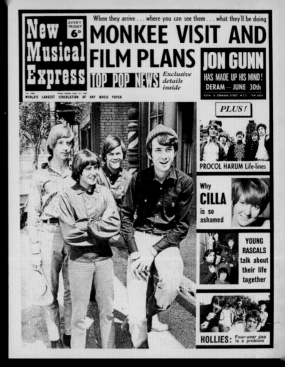

waterline. Scratching the surface even a little would reveal an undercurrent of youth activity that did not always find its way into the upper echelons of the charts: mods vs rockers. They hated one another with a passion (despite owning different models of motorbikes). The mods thought rockers were dirty, unkempt and outmoded; the rockers thought the mods effeminate and vain.

The choice of separate venues for their weekend gatherings meant that, more often than not, trouble was avoided. However, when the locations clashed, a major conflagration was unavoidable. Most affected of all were the

British seaside resorts, which drew thousands of tourists for the traditional Bank Holiday weekend getaway. Unfortunately, neither mods nor rockers were about to share generously, and the rampaging soon spread from Margate, in Kent, to Brighton, in East Sussex: no picturesque resort seemed safe. The year 1964 witnessed a particular concentration of coastal clashes, with pitched battles on the beaches and inside the seafront hotels and bars.

The events were front-page news and a genuinely scary development for the middle classes. However, within eighteen months, the newspapers had tired of reporting the violence, and the culture clash disappeared from the front pages.

By the latter half of the decade, the growing popularity of 'flower power' and the so-called 'Summer of Love' – as the media dubbed 1967 – made the mods versus rockers fights seem a dim and distant memory. As British music veered off towards rock, with bands such as The Who breaking through, American influences returned to infect UK youth culture.

The Haight-Ashbury scene in San Francisco was one geographical hub of the flower-power scene; and LSD was the drug at its nucleus. With the trend towards greater communal awareness came a sea change in fashion, with kaftan coats, coloured sunglasses and all manner of extravagant and ethnic hippie clothes. This counterculture movement dominated much of the late '60s and – although driven initially by a socio-political thirst for change – eventually became so consumed by mainstream culture that it represented little more than a fashionable whim. Numerous artists found fresh popularity among the legions of bare-footed festival-goers, including Sonny and Cher (see No. 16) and Simon & Garfunkel (see No. 53).

The dawn of the '70s saw a cultural hangover from the '60s, with the deaths of Jimi Hendrix, Janis Joplin and Jim Morrison providing a tragic advertisement for the previous decade's excess. Nonetheless, the '60s must be acknowledged as one of the most fruitful and innovative decades in modern history.

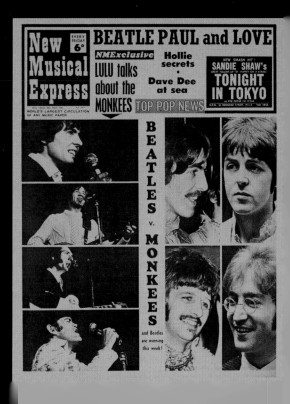

37 The Power Of Love
Jennifer Rush

Release Date: 29.06.85
No. Weeks In Chart: 36
Reached No. 1: 12.10.85
Total Sales: 1,321,530

The first UK million-seller by a female artist and 1985's biggest record came from the American-born wonder-lungs of Jennifer Rush.

The first UK million-seller by a female artist, 'The Power of Love' is a wedding reception favourite and karaoke singer's nightmare. Born Heidi Stern in New York City to an opera singer father and pianist mother, Jennifer Rush adopted her stage name in 1983 and her wonder-lungs helped her career take off soon after.

Although this was the biggest UK seller of 1985, the original release failed to make the Top 40 across the Atlantic in Rush's homeland – although the Celine Dion version went all the way to the US top spot in 1994.

A Spanish-language version of the track, 'Si Tu Eres Mi Hombre Y Yo Tu Mujer', was a No. 1 success in Spain. Subsequent albums, singles and tours have consistently sold heavily (in 1987, a Jennifer Rush album was second only to U2's watershed behemoth *The Joshua Tree* in American sales).

High-profile duets with Elton John, Michael Bolton and Placido Domingo, as well as contributions to Disney soundtracks, illustrate that Rush was far from a fleeting success.

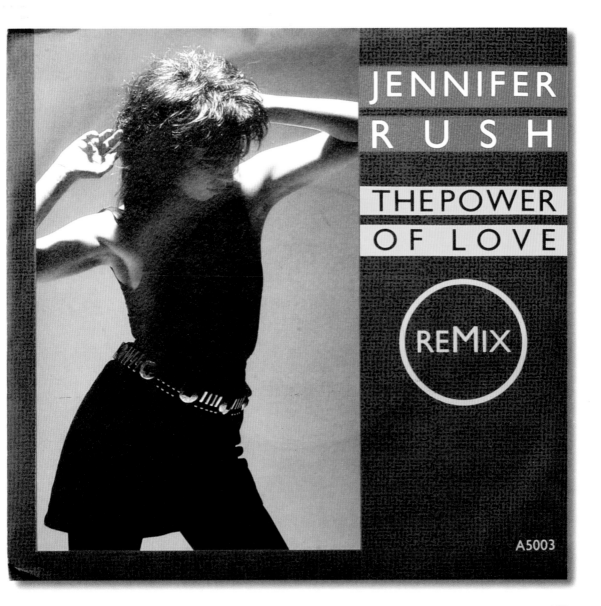

38 Unchained Melody
Gareth Gates

Release Date: 30.03.02
No. Weeks In Chart: 27
Reached No. 1: 30.03.02
Total Sales: 1,318,714

This song became a debut million-seller for the people's champion in the rush to be crowned Pop Idol.

Amazingly, this is the second entry for this song on the chart (see No. 9). This single sent Gates straight in at No. 1 amid a frenzy of hyper-ventilating teenage girls. A shy and gangly 17-year-old from Bradford, Gareth Gates captured the hearts of the watching millions when his severe stutter made him take over 25 seconds to introduce himself to the panel of *Pop Idol* judges.

When Gates then proceeded to sing a polished version of a track by his favourite band, Westlife, for many people the race to find a Pop Idol was over. Although he struggled midway through the series, Gates returned to form and was only narrowly pipped to the post by surprise winner Will Young (see No. 12).

Yet while Will Young was soon working with Burt Bacharach and discussing his jazz and soul influences, former student Gates cited Westlife and Cliff Richard as his two inspirations. His squeaky-clean image and supposedly saccharine personality were derided by the media, but in no way damaged his chart success. Although criticised by the more cynical elements of the music business for – potentially – lacking longevity, Gates is said to have earned

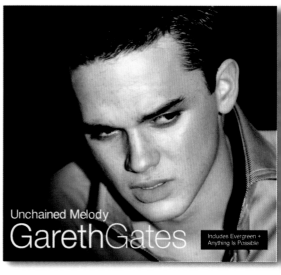

Unchained Melody
GarethGates
Includes Evergreen + Anything Is Possible

over £3 million in the twelve months since the *Pop Idol* programme.

The success shows no signs of drying up just yet. Gates and Young combined to score a joint No. 1 in late 2002 with their cover of The Beatles' 'The Long and Winding Road'. And Gates' version of 'Unchained Melody' has to date clocked up 27 weeks in the chart – but in October 2002 was still selling . . .

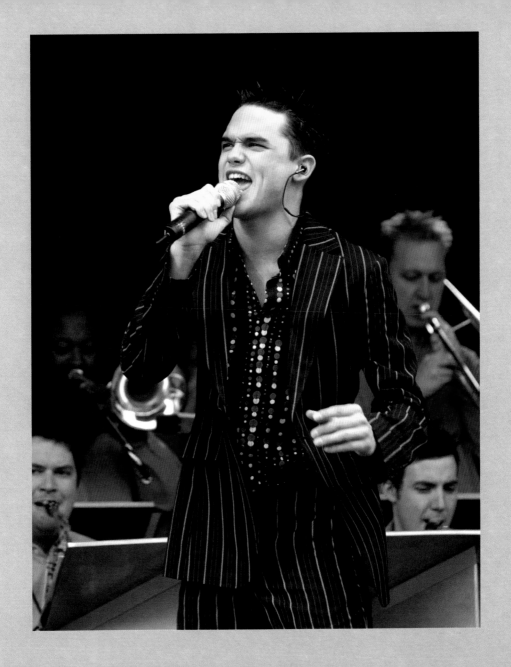

39 My Heart Will Go On
Celine Dion

Release Date: 21.02.98
No. Weeks In Chart: 20
Reached No. 1: 21.02.98
Total Sales: 1,312,551

The Celine Dion version was nearly omitted from the final cut of *Titanic*, as producer James Cameron refused initially to include any vocal pieces in the film.

One of the list's genuine global super-songs, 'My Heart Will Go On' provided French-Canadian mega-chanteuse Celine Dion with a new pinnacle of mind-boggling commercial success. This lead song from the soundtrack of *Titanic* was almost as omnipresent as the biggest-grossing film of all time.

The Dion version – now synonymous with that blockbuster movie – nearly didn't make it to the final cut, as producer James Cameron strongly resisted the move to include vocal songs in the film. Eventually, songwriter James Horner added lyrics to his instrumental 'love theme' and, with surprising simplicity, Dion and her husband Rene released the original demo version of the tune.

Alternative versions of the song soon began to appear, with record label Sony themselves releasing an array of variations, including an album cut, a soundtrack cut, an edited version with movie dialogue and even a dance version.

However, it was the original Dion rendition that broke the records. In 1998 alone, the song was heard by in excess of 100 million radio

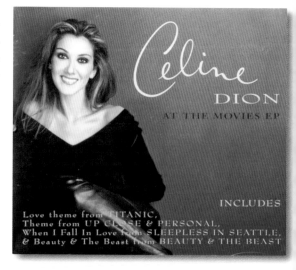

listeners worldwide. Suitably pragmatic – although hardly straight-talking – when asked about the repetitive consequences of this track on her live shows of the future, Celine offered the comment, 'It's not like a song or a movie, it's like a magic moment, so I don't mind to sing it over and over again.'

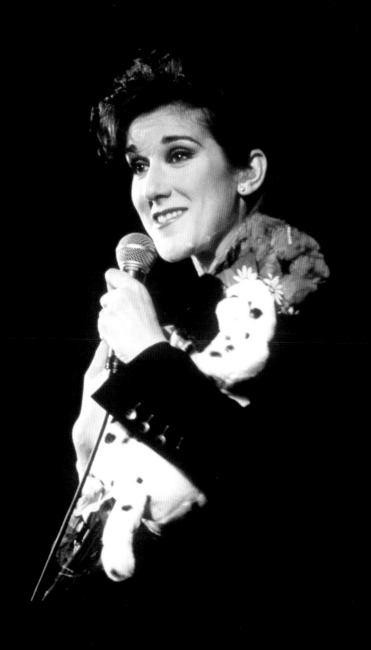

40 Wannabe
Spice Girls

Release Date: 20.07.96
No. Weeks In Chart: 26
Reached No. 1: 27.07.96
Total Sales: 1,269,841

The powerful combination of the girls' exaggerated personas and gang-like mentality – dubbed by one reporter as 'Oasis with a Wonderbra' – seized the headlines from the previously all-conquering boy bands.

The epitome of the juggernaut that would become 'girl power', this debut single was a brash statement of intent, which some critics scorned and even compared to a nursery rhyme. Yet it was a new entry at No. 1 and the year's best-seller.

Others were puzzled by the 'zig-a-zig-ah's' that punctuated the lyrics – the first of many new words that the Spice Girls have since added to the modern lexicon. Even the advert that the girls responded to in *The Stage* asked openly for five 'wannabe starlets' to form a band. Unlike Hear'Say (see No. 65), only 400 hopefuls applied. The fizzing single was supported by a one-take video shot at King's Cross-St Pancras station, which showcased the girls' 'full-on' characters.

Seizing the headlines from boy bands Take That and Boyzone, 'Wannabe' ousted Gary Barlow from the top spot and went on to reach No. 1 in a further 21 countries worldwide. The girls – branded Baby, Posh, Scary, Ginger and Sporty by *Smash Hits* magazine – had seemingly reinvented every rule in the pop universe and, from now on, things would never be the same. Within a mere eighteen months of signing their first record deal, the Spice Girls were the biggest band on the planet.

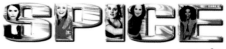

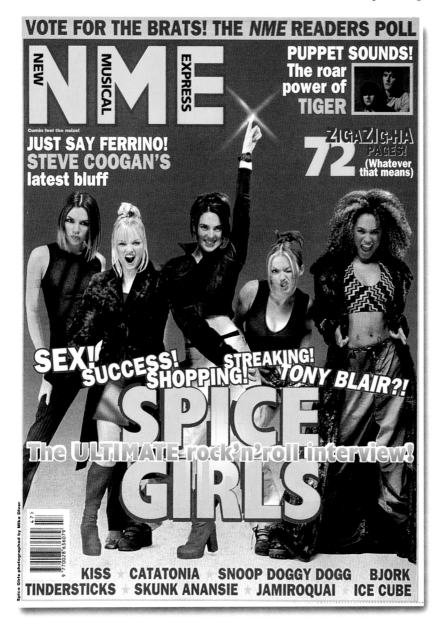

VOTE FOR THE BRATS! THE *NME* READERS POLL

NEW MUSICAL EXPRESS

NME

Cumin feel the noize!

PUPPET SOUNDS!
The roar power of TIGER

JUST SAY FERRINO!
STEVE COOGAN'S latest bluff

ZIGAZIG-HA
72 PAGES!
(Whatever that means)

SEX! SUCCESS! SHOPPING! STREAKING! TONY BLAIR?!

SPICE
GIRLS

The ULTIMATE rock'n'roll interview!

Spice Girls photographed by Mike Diver

KISS ★ CATATONIA ★ SNOOP DOGGY DOGG ★ BJORK
TINDERSTICKS ★ SKUNK ANANSIE ★ JAMIROQUAI ★ ICE CUBE

41 Killing Me Softly
Fugees

Release Date: 8.06.96
No. Weeks In Chart: 20
Reached No. 1: 8.06.96
Total Sales: 1,268,157

The song's acoustic funkiness and musical directness provided a refreshing blast of simplicity that turned the world of hip-hop on its head.

This hip-hop version of the 1973 Roberta Flack classic was the Fugees' breakthrough single. The song was the perfect showcase for the band's manifesto pledge to return hip-hop to its musical roots, concerned as they were about the increasingly stereotyped – and at times violent – machismo of the mainstream version of the genre. The vocal prowess of Lauryn Hill, MC skills of Pras and production brilliance of Wyclef Jean made this one of the stand-out tracks of 1996.

Wyclef is the son of a preacher, his cousin Pras the son of a deacon, both Haitian immigrants living in Brooklyn. The latter was a schoolmate of Lauryn Hill; together they formed the New Jersey-based Tranzlator Crew, producing songs from their basement studio.

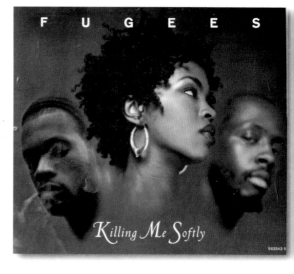

A name change to the symbolic Fugees led to modest underground success with their debut album *Blunted On Reality*. However, it was this single and the accompanying album, *The Score*, which turned the band into megastars – both records were Grammy-winners and No. 1s in the US and around the globe. Hill described the hit album, which drew on a multitude of influences, including hip-hop, rap, reggae, Caribbean and R&B, as 'an audio film'. A follow-up album has been persistently delayed, as all three have enjoyed successful solo careers. Hill (who was still at Columbia University when this song took off) continues to pursue a parallel acting career.

THE FUGEES
Killing Me Softly *(Columbia)*

ALSO SUFFERING follow-up
fever are Haitian-born,
American chartbeating rappers
The Fugees, who've opted to
ransack the Roberta Flack back
catalogue for a suitable riposte
to the justified success of their
'Fu-Gee-La' single. Gone are the
cunning hip-hop twists and
turns, replaced by mounds of
sugary gospel. Where classic De
La Soul vibes used to meet R&B,
a Tina-Turner-does-*Songs Of
Praise* and a comedy sitar fight
for attention.
    The Fugees can, have and will
do better than this barber shop
bollocks, so perhaps it's best if
we just forget it ever happened,
eh?

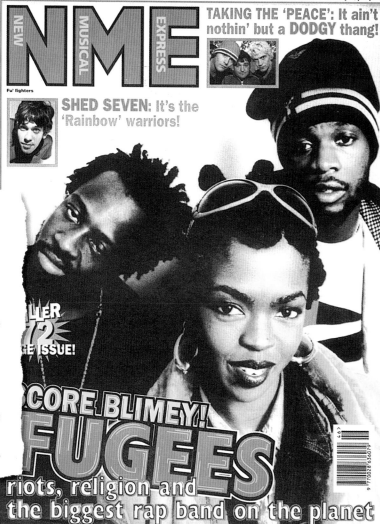

16 November 1996   90p S(US)3.95

NME
NEW MUSICAL EXPRESS

Fu' fighters

TAKING THE 'PEACE': It ain't
nothin' but a **DODGY** thang!

SHED SEVEN: It's the
'Rainbow' warriors!

LLER
72
E ISSUE!

CORE BLIMEY!
FUGEES
riots, religion and
the biggest rap band on the planet

TRICKY ★ SCREAMING TREES ★ GORKY'S ZYGOTIC MYNCI
EAST 17 ★ JOHNNY CASH ★ *MICHAEL COLLINS* ★ KENICKIE

42 Never Ever
All Saints

Release Date: 22.11.97

No. Weeks In Chart: 24

Reached No. 1: 17.01.98

Total Sales: 1,254,604

The steamy melancholy of a jilted lover that was 'Never Ever' was the epitome of the All Saints' style.

With the Spice Girls having reinvented the world of pop and already five No. 1 hits into their pivotal career, record companies the world over were scouring for the next big girl band. Many observers touted All Saints as exactly that, especially after their debut as a quartet reached the Top Five.

The band were, in fact, anything but the next Spices. After a faltering start on ZTT (see No.'s 7 and 22) and the departure of one original member, Melanie Blatt and Shaznay Lewis recruited two Canadian-born sisters, Nicole and Natalie Appleton, following a chance meeting between Mel's taxi-driver father and the younger Appleton, Nicole.

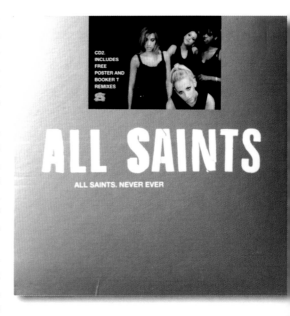

Sultry looks, accomplished soulful and blues-inflected vocals and a darker lyrical subject matter all compounded to broaden the All Saints' appeal beyond the teen market. The second single was a slow burner, only hitting the top slot after ten weeks of release, but symbolically bumping the Spice Girls' 'Spice Up Your Life' off No. 1.

Sophisticated cover versions ('Under The Bridge') blended in well with funky sassy originals ('Bootie Call') to reinforce the girls' burgeoning reputation as the 'thinking-man's' girl band. Unfortunately, relations within the group were always somewhat fraught and it thus came as little surprise to the record-buying public when the break-up of All Saints was announced in 2001 – after a chart career consisting entirely of Top Ten hits.

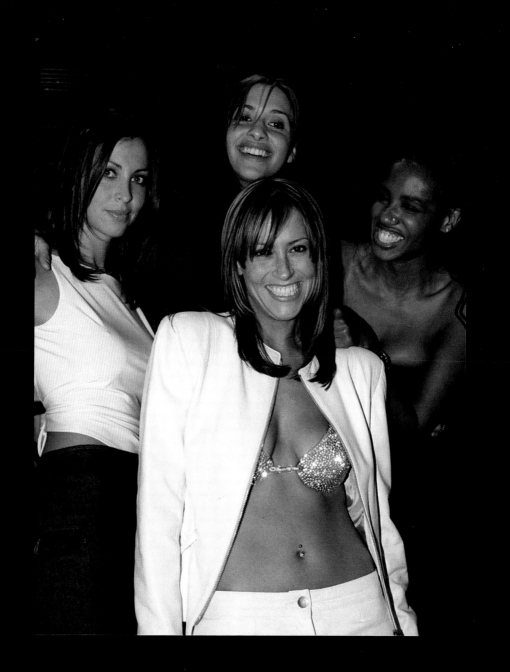

Boy Bands

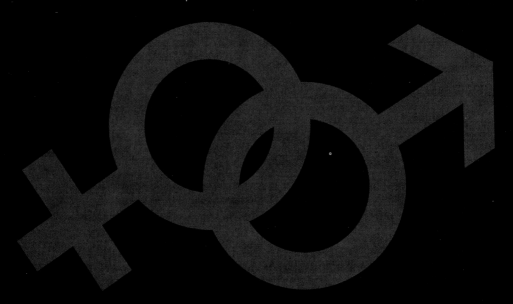

Girl Groups

When Take That split up in 1996, it seemed to thousands of teenage girls that the end of the world was nigh.

It was bad enough that Robbie had already left, plunging into an abyss of drink, drugs, weight gain and bad hair. The fans sought solace from the hope that even if Robbie was consigned to the history books as an inevitable future chart failure, at least there was Gary Barlow's solo career to look forward to (see No. 98).

Manufactured bands are a part of music history – fact. Few sectors of the music industry attract so much scorn and fewer still sell as many records. All-female jazz and dance bands

had existed in the 1920s, but after World War II there was a proliferation of girl groups – both African-American and white – centred mostly on the swing genre.

However, the consensus is that the first girl group was the Chantels in 1958, fronted by Arlene Smith who sang on their hit single 'Maybe'. The first US No. 1 hit by such a line-up came three years later, with the Shirelles' 'Will You Love Me Tomorrow'. The early '60s was the first true era of girl bands, with acts such as the Marvelettes, the Cookies and the Chiffons all enjoying success. Almost all were black, hailing from America, often very young – usually teenagers – and often talented gospel singers.

Studio producers would blend a great song with a great set of voices, although new band line-ups were sometimes kept anonymous for fear of alienating the white record-buying public. From this era came such big hits as The Crystals' 'Da Doo Ron Ron' and the Marvelettes' 'Please Mr Postman'. Even back then, certain formulas were at work. Four different girl bands – the Spandells, the Secrets, Bettye Swann and Terri Stevens – all released different songs with the same title, 'The Boy Next Door'.

The Shangri-Las were one of the first white female bands, with hits such as 'Leader of the Pack' and 'You Can't Go Home Anymore'; with their leather-clad image and frequent radio bans, they were also one of the first to court controversy. Of course, this period also witnessed girl groups with much more to offer than bland formula. The Supremes were the

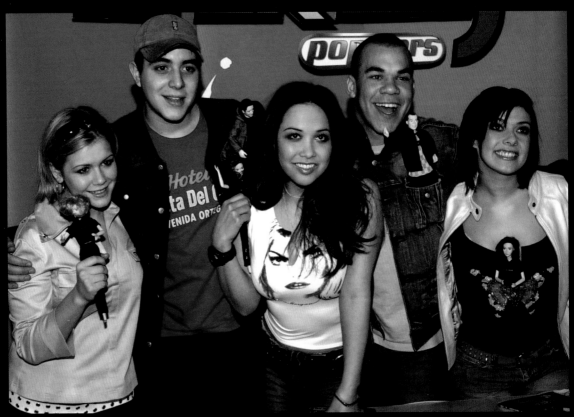

obvious example, with their sophisticated image and quality song-writing team of Holland, Holland and Lamont. Other writers who have written for girl bands include Neil Sedaka, Neil Diamond, Paul Simon and Brian Wilson.

The boys weren't long in following. There had been all-male quality pop acts already – the Ink Spots and The Temptations, for example – but The Monkees were perhaps the clearest case of a manufactured band. Recruited for a television show, the group's music was not even played by the band members, yet their popularity was huge. Although intended as a television rival to The Beatles' Hard Days Night, The Monkees still managed to retain an air of credibility. Later boy band incarnations have seen acts such as The Osmonds, The Bay City Rollers, Bros and even Wham!

Leapfrog ahead to the mid-'90s: Bananarama still hold the title of Britain's biggest-ever girl band; Take That have split and Boyzone have stepped into the fray, seemingly unchallenged

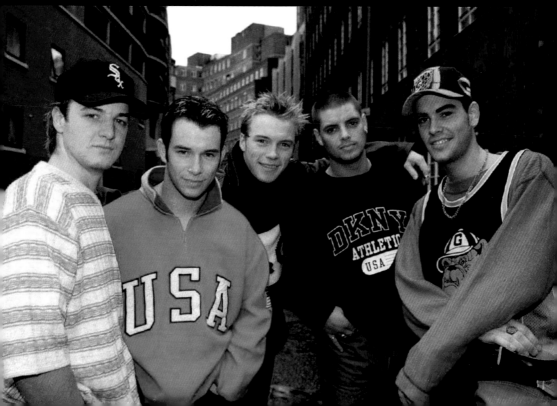

hen came Spice World. Within months, we were besieged by Posh, Scary, Baby, Sporty and Ginger: 'girl power' had arrived. Their cleverly constructed image combined sex appeal with flashings of self-confidence, and boy did it work (see No.'s 40 and 67). In the wake of the semi-retirement of the Spices, it was Steps who took an unlikely hold of the pop market, with their Abba-esque hits and TV-friendly dance routines; their gender mix proved a popular twist on the manufactured band, and made them the biggest-grossing tour act of 2000.

Of course, in true manufactured band fashion, behind every great act there is a great svengali. The late, great Phil Spector was lurking in the shadows behind acts such as The Crystals and The Ronettes. Motown helped mould many a top girl band, and Lou Perlman can claim to have brought us both the Backstreet Boys and N*Sync.

Legend has it that Perlman used to run a charter airline company and would regularly take highly lucrative bookings from New Kids on the Block, at the time the world's biggest act. (NKOTB were themselves a follow-on act for mega-producer and former New Edition maestro Maurice Starr.) Realising he could make more money from managing these boy bands than from managing their aeroplanes, Perlman changed career.

British manufactured bands have at times made their managers as famous as them – take, for example, pop impresarios such as Simon Fuller (the Spice Girls), Nigel Martin-Smith (Take That), Tom Watkins (East 17) and Louis Walsh (Boyzone, Westlife).

Critical scepticism may highlight each band's lack of songwriting ability (Elvis or Cliff anyone?), their frequent recruitment through auditions (*NME* classifieds?), the incessant managerial input (Peter Grant, Brian Epstein), the expensive videos (Michael Jackson has been known to spend the odd . . . erm . . . penny) and their eventual ventures into far less successful solo careers (The Beatles, Queen, The Rolling Stones . . .). Of course, no one claims that A1 have left a greater cultural and social impact than the Fab Four (at least I hope not).

However, next time you grab the remote control to switch over hastily from yet another boy or girl band on heavy rotation on MTV, think again. Britney Spears spent longer singing as an unsigned act before breaking through than Travis did. N*Sync once played 250 gigs in one year, a record of which even Bruce Springsteen would be proud.

The commercial pressure on such bands is mightily oppressive – when Backstreet Boys' *Black and Blue* album only sold eight million copies, whispers of a 'flop' bizarrely began to circulate. Almost all boy and girl band members suffer exhaustion at some point, from schedules they may have little or no control over. Plus, someone out there likes it . . . When N*Sync released their album *No Strings Attached*, the previous *Billboard* record for first-week sales was 1.1 million copies (held by boy band rivals The Backstreet Boys). However, N*Sync shifted that in ten hours. By the end of the first week, they'd sold 2.4 million units.

Maybe you were so cool that at the age of twelve you were clutching a gatefold sleeve copy of a rare Velvet Underground album; but most people cannot claim such pre-teen vision. They want to be served up with 'a boyish one', 'a wacky one', 'a dull-but-good-at-music-one', 'a dancing (and possibly gay) one' and 'an older-one-for-the-mums'.

Scratch beneath the 'manufactured' surface of any formula band, and you will find an almost archetypal career path plotted out. Early gigs in gay cabaret; the breakthrough single; tabloid frenzy; tours, possible feature film; rumours of band problems; one member leaves, sales start to slip; solo careers are mooted but no way are they going to split – they split. Surprise.

Each time a member announces that he/she is: (a) leaving; (b) gay; (c) really a rocker at heart; or, (d) disillusioned with the artistic and subsequent psychosexual confines of the pop/dance genre, lesser chart acts breathe a sigh of relief and schedule in their next single.

Then the doom-mongers waiting in the wings herald the final (and oh-so deserved) death knell of the manufactured band and rush to announce the return of 'real' music.

Until the next time . . .

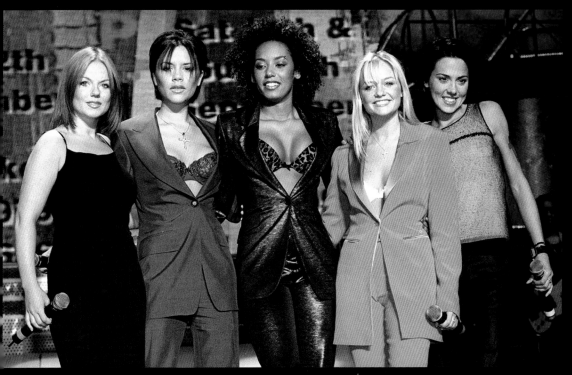

43 Gangsta's Paradise
Coolio Featuring LV

Release Date: 28.10.95
No. Weeks In Chart: 20
Reached No. 1: 28.10.95
Total Sales: 1,246,306

Legend has it that after some initial reluctance to the idea, Stevie Wonder heard the track and faxed back his approval the very same afternoon.

This Grammy-winning track was built around a sample from Stevie Wonder's 1976 tune 'Pastime Paradise'. A seductive yet dark lament about inner-city desperation, delivered alongside the gospel vocals of LV and a full choir, Coolio claimed to have undergone a spiritual experience when writing the track with his old friend LV, who himself later recorded his own version as a B-side to his 'Throw Your Hands Up' single.

The song was on the worldwide No. 1 soundtrack to the movie *Dangerous Minds*, based on the true story of former marine LouAnne Johnson's life teaching English to under-privileged inner city kids at a North Californian High School. Her book, *My Posse Don't Do Homework*, was a best-seller.

Coolio was born Artis Leon Ivey, Jr. He took his name after being ribbed for looking like 'Coolio Iglesias'. This Compton, LA-born rapper was one of that city's earliest rap exponents. Nonetheless, Coolio enjoyed only sporadic initial success; less glamorous moments including a stint as a forestry fireman.

This song was his UK chart peak, the biggest seller of 1995 and a No. 1 success in the US and all across Europe. This was the first time a hardcore rapper had taken the UK's No. 1 position, an event described by one reporter as 'quite spectacular'.

Although it is the track for which Coolio is best remembered, the hard-hitting 'Gangsta's Paradise' was by no means typical of the rapper's material. Previous singles such as 'Fantastic Voyage' were characterised by humourous lyrics and playful videos. Record label Tommy Boy were initially concerned that the altogether darker 'Gangsta's Paradise' would alienate Coolio fans, and convinced the rapper to leave the track off his album. It was only after it appeared on the *Dangerous Minds* soundtrack, that the song really took off.

Father to seven children, Coolio once described himself as 'a ghetto witch doctor'. He has also appeared in scores of films and television shows, including *Batman & Robin*, and achieved the second-highest score ever on US-TV show *Pictionary*.

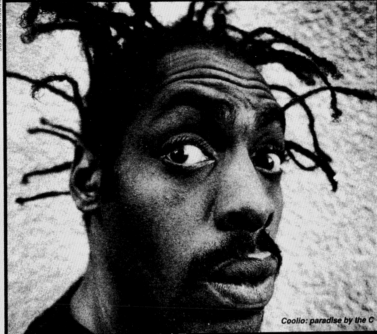

Coolio: paradise by the C

SINGLE OF THE WEEK

COOLIO FEATURING LV
Gangsta's Paradise *(Tommy Boy)*

WILL THE circle of murderous violence, bad education, poverty traps, unemployment and dilapidated housing remain forever unbroken in America's ghettos? Coolio sees only hopelessness, with no option of deliverance or redemption for the besieged youth except in death.

His missive from the frontlines of a racially fractured America, rent asunder by militias and devious politicians, greed and addiction, points out the essential nihilism of the gangsta condition. And what a breathtaking, doleful and melancholy record 'Gangsta's Paradise' is.

The most visible rapper currently extant and his singing sidekick, LV, puts an acetylene torch to Stevie Wonder's 'Pastime Paradise' and constructs something new from its ashes… Stabbing strings, a keyboard drone, a massed gothic chorus of gospel voices and a beat ticking time to the bitter end, are all weaved together into this solemn theme tune, hijacked from the soundtrack to the Michelle Pfeiffer vehicle *Dangerous Minds*.

'Gangsta's Paradise' is akin to LL Cool J's 'Crossroads', three years on – only more apocalyptic. And, in the wake of Time Warner's unfortunate decision to ditch Interscope Records (and hence silence Death Row Records, Nine Inch Nails and a host of supposedly 'morally dubious' acts), a scary precedent has been set, which this single defies. Without a single swear word.

44 Diana
Paul Anka

Release Date: 9.08.57

No. Weeks In Chart: 25

Reached No. 1: 30.08.57

Total Sales: 1,240,000

Heavily influenced by Chuck Berry and Fats Domino, Anka's musical technicality blended seamlessly with lashings of romance to garner huge commercial success.

Fifteen-year-old Canadian schoolboy Paul Anka penned this love song in tribute to Diana Ayoub, his younger sibling's babysitter who was five years his senior. The following year, aged only sixteen, he won a trip to New York by collecting soup labels – within four months of arriving in the Big Apple, he had a US and UK No. 1 song with 'Diana', which went on to sell 20 million copies, spending nine weeks at the UK's top slot (bumping the King's 'All Shook Up' off the top).

Promptly launched as the youngest crooning star of the '50s, Anka was, however, no mere pretty face – his songwriting accolades outstrip even his mammoth chart career. He went on to arrange songs for Buddy Holly, write the lyrics to Sinatra's 'My Way' and pen hits for Tom Jones and Donny Osmond in a career which boasts over 900 songs and 123 albums to date. He also wrote the theme tune to the mega-popular TV show *The Tonight Show Starring Johnny Carson*.

This former teenage talent show impersonator earned seven UK Top Ten hits, but this record is dwarfed by his US achievements of endlessly sold-out casino shows and 42 million sales. In 1963, this son of Lebanese immigrants released 'Remember Diana', a sequel to his breakthrough hit. He is one of that rare group of artists who have enjoyed chart success over five decades, ensuring over 90 million performances of his songs along the way.

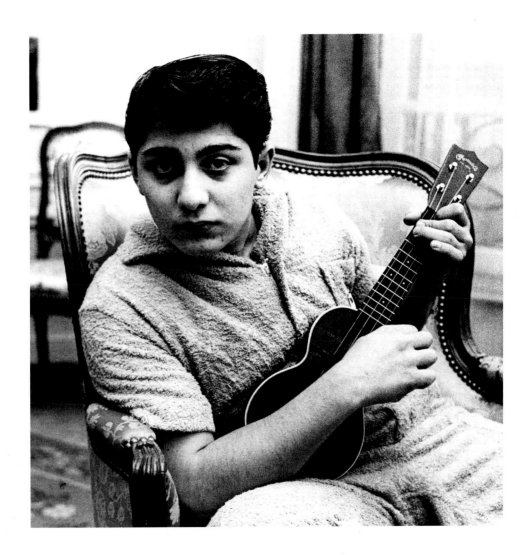

45 Think Twice
Celine Dion

Release Date: 22.10.94
No. Weeks In Chart: 31
Reached No. 1: 4.02.95
Total Sales: 1,234,982

The hugely successful Celine Dion has now racked up worldwide sales in excess of 120 million albums.

'Think Twice' was written by the English songwriting duo of Andy Hill and Pete Sinfield. The latter was an ex-roadie and lyricist for '60s prog-rock juggernaut King Crimson who had also penned 'Heart Of Stone' for Cher (see also No. 16).

Released in the same year as her *Billboard*-topping cover version of Jennifer Rush's 'The Power of Love' (see No. 37), this was yet another commercial mega-hit for the former Eurovision song contest winner.

'Think Twice' was at the UK top spot for five weeks at the same time as it was No. 1 in America. The English-language album *The Colour Of My Love*, from which this track was taken, was a pivotal release for Dion, as it contained – in the liner notes – the surprise declaration of her love for, and previously concealed relationship with, her manager and mentor, Rene Angelil, who was said to have wept uncontrollably when he first read the announcement. And not for the first time . . .

Dion recorded her first self-composition at the age of twelve, and sent it to Angelil. When she later sang for him in his office, the manager was so overcome . . . that he burst into tears.

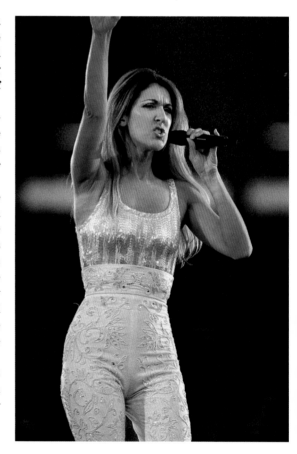

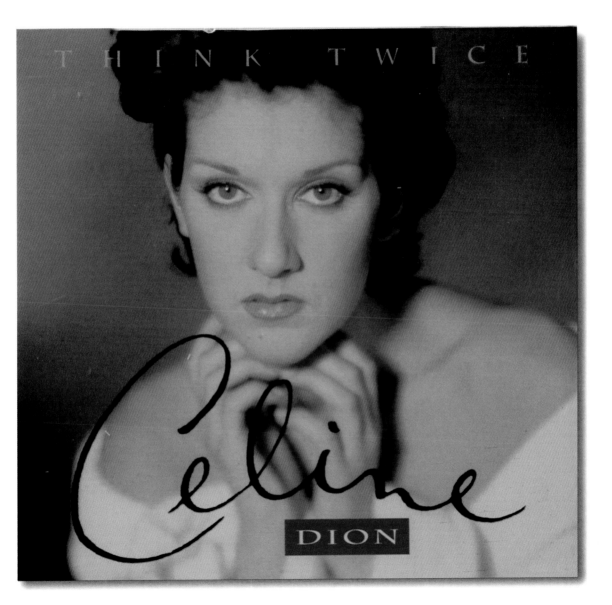

46 It's Now Or Never
Elvis Presley

Release Date: 3.11.60
No. Weeks In Chart: 21
Reached No. 1: 3.11.60
Total Sales: 1,210,000

The King's biggest ever hit in the UK and – remarkably for an artist with over one billion global record sales – the only song to feature in this list.

This cod-operatic ballad was an Americanised version of the 1899 Neapolitan standard, 'O Sole Mio'. The song represented a seismic shift in musical direction for the former hip-swivelling rock 'n' roller. Copyright wrangles in the UK initially threatened to delay the release for seven years, but once these legal issues were resolved, the British (and American) public bought this single in huge quantities. Elvis' fifth No. 1 entered the UK charts at the top with first-week sales hitting the 750,000 mark; a million copies were sold within 40 days. It stayed at the summit for eight weeks.

This was Elvis' second single since leaving the army and is seen by many experts as a song caught between two distinct phases – sandwiched between the 'classic' era of his early Sun/RCA recordings and the rather less critically favoured film and soundtrack work of the '60s. Nonetheless, this song started a run of nine consecutive UK chart-toppers, which were only stifled when dwindling credibility and the arrival of Merseybeat eroded his chart popularity. It is worth noting that, by 1966, Decca Records had four singles that had sold one million copies (see also No.'s 31, 47 and 51).

'It's Now Or Never' came at a frantic time for the King: he had left the army in early 1960 to find two tons of fanmail waiting for him; the charts were enjoying a trad-jazz phase (see No. 58) and instrumental groups like The Shadows were also hugely popular; he had started dating Priscilla Beaulieu; his manager and former travelling showman, Colonel Tom Parker, would shortly put a price of $150,000 a gig on his head; and his film *G.I. Blues* was grossing $190,000 a night.

It was only four years since RCA had launched their new signing, described as 'a wild and turbulent rock and roller' and in that time he had taken over the hearts and minds of the teenage world. Unfortunately, his schedule of three films a year soon took his focus away

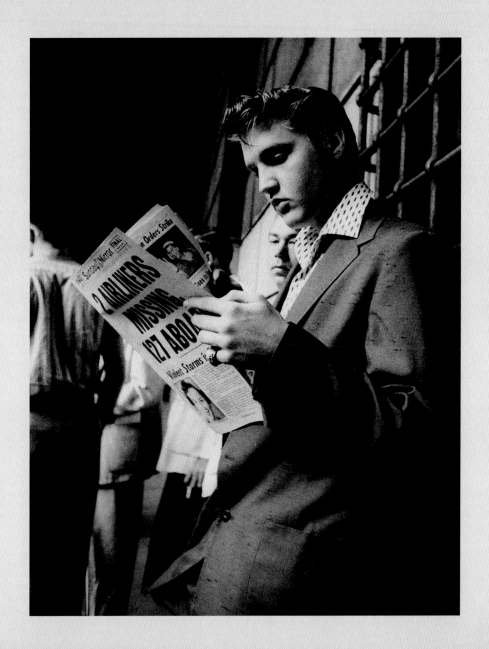

from his core passion for music, leaving patient fans to wait until his 1968 comeback for a famous return to form.

In June 2002 – 25 years after his death – the King (billed as Elvis vs JXL) enjoyed a record-breaking return to No.1 with a remix of an obscure B-side, 'A Little Less Conversation'. This soundtrack to the Nike World Cup advertising campaign gave Elvis his 18th No. 1 in the UK, a feat unmatched even by The Beatles, and one coming an astonishing 25 years after his last UK chart-topper.

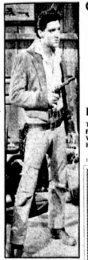

GOLD DISC IN DOUBLE QUICK TIME—

Presley's 'Now Or Never' breaks all speed records for sales!

DEALERS OVERWHELMED BY CROWDS DEMANDING DISC

ELVIS PRESLEY—THE UNDOUBTED KING OF RECORD STARS. THAT IS HOW HIS LATEST BRITISH DISC TRIUMPH HAS BEEN HAILED. THE SALES IN THIS COUNTRY OF "IT'S NOW OR NEVER" HAVE BEEN FASTER THAN ANY PREVIOUS HIT ANYWHERE IN THE WORLD. IT IS VIRTUALLY CERTAIN HE WILL GET A GOLD DISC WITHIN A MONTH OF ISSUE—HIS FIRST FROM BRITISH SALES ALONE.

Less than two weeks after it had been released, sales exceeded three-quarters of a million and the waxing is selling in such quantity that by early next week, demand could have boosted sales to a million!

Presley broke all records with an advanced order of more than 548,000 for the disc by its issue on October 28.

On Wednesday of this week, just twelve days later, Decca, who distribute Presley's label RCA, had received orders from dealers for 771,100 copies.

One dealer in a London suburb reported selling twelve times more copies of "It's Now Or Never" than any other disc last Saturday.

Another, in an effort to cope with the fantastic crowds thronging his shop for two hours, only admitted those who wanted the Presley disc.

The previous fastest-selling disc was Harry Belafonte's "Mary's Boy Child" (another RCA issue) which between mid-October and December, 1957, sold a million copies in this country alone.

ADAM FAITH IN ABC-TV PANTO

ADAM FAITH will be one of the stars in ABC-TV's spectacular Christmas afternoon pantomime, "Alice Through The Looking Box." He is among a host of new names issued this week for the programme—which is still not fully cast.

As forecast, Jeannie Carson will also take part—in the title role. The NME two weeks ago told in the NME two weeks ago that includes Harry Secombe, David Hughes, Pete Murray, Joe Henderson and the Vernons Girls.

The time slot set for the hour-

first picture of ELVIS PRESLEY in his next picture, "Flaming Star," in which he plays a part-Indian. His role calls for gunplay and fist fighting.

SHADOWS TOP LONG 1961 TOUR

A LONG one-night stand tour is being lined up early next year for the Shadows as a starring attraction in their own right—to cover major theatre and cinema circuits.

The tour has been made possible by Cliff Richard's considerable film commitments at the beginning of next year.

As Cliff's plans have not yet been finalised, it is therefore impossible for Howes to arrange an itinerary for the Shadows at this stage, but it is expected that they will play one-nighters for a minimum of eight weeks.

When Cliff's film has been completed, the Shadows will rejoin him for further variety and one-night dates. There is no question of the Cliff-Shadows separation being a permanent one, the group's manager, Peter Gormley, told the NME.

Cliff Richard star of New Year's Eve show

CLIFF RICHARD will headline ATV's "Saturday Spectacular" on New Year's Eve. This is the latest development following a change...

JUDY WON'T LET MANCHESTER DOWN

THE "Evening With Judy Garland" concert at Manchester Free Trade Hall, which had to be cancelled last month, is being rearranged for...

CONNIE FRANCIS GETS NME POLL CUP ON U.S. TV

CONNIE FRANCIS is the first of the 1960 NME poll-winning artists to be presented with a trophy. Millions of Americans will see Connie with it on a major TV programme.

Her trophy, a cup—for being voted World's Outstanding Female Singer—was rushed to America last weekend so that it could be presented on the show.

The programme—"Person To Person," in which the subject is questioned by interviewer Charles Collingwood—is one of America's major documentary series.

It was being telerecorded by CBS in New York yesterday (Thursday) for showing throughout America during January.

London's 'Music Man' confirmed

HOLLYWOOD screen star Van Johnson returns to the stage in the London production of "The Music Man," one of Broadway's most successful musicals.

The signing announced on Wednesday, was forecast in the NME last summer.

The show, which will be staged at the Adelphi in the spring, was written by Meredith Wilson.

POP STARS AT BALL

'It was only four years since RCA had launched their new signing, described as "a wild and turbulent rock and roller" and in that time he had taken over the hearts and minds of the teenage world.'

NEW MUSICAL EXPRESS

THANK YOU NME READERS FOR AGAIN MAKING THIS A VERY HAPPY TIME

FOR ME STOP I ALWAYS SEEM TO BE AWAY WHEN I GET SOME GOOD NEWS

STOP MUCH LOVE TO YOU ALL FROM HOMESICK DUSTY.

L CYA14Ø INTL CULVER CITY CALIF 23 2 138PPST

LT EDITOR NEWMUSEX

   LONDON(ENGLAND)

FRIENDS STOP HIGHLY HONORED AND PLEASED WITH POLL RESULTS AM

MOST GRATEFUL TO ALL WARMEST WISHES FOR HAPPY HOLIDAYS

   ELVIS.

47 Green, Green Grass Of Home
Tom Jones

Release Date: 10.11.66

No. Weeks In Chart: 22

Reached No. 1: 1.12.66

Total Sales: 1,205,000

When this single was released, Elvis Presley is said to have spent hours phoning radio stations to request the song.

This song helped to reinforce Jones' position as a transatlantic star in the '60s but, surprisingly, it is only his second and final No. 1 to date. The son of a coal miner (and himself a former door-to-door vacuum-cleaner salesman), Jones' career took off overnight when his second single, 'It's Not Unusual', reached No. 1. Radio One initially refused to play Jones' material, citing it as too raunchy, but pirate radio stations such as Radio Caroline championed him instead.

Early radio plays of his songs led many American listeners to believe that Jones was black – his baritone-to-tenor range was famously admired by Elvis Presley (later to become a close friend), who warmed up for his own shows by singing 'Delilah'.

Alongside balladeer Engelbert Humperdinck (both men were managed by the late Gordon Mills), Jones went on to enjoy enormous success Stateside, carving out a niche that was in direct contrast to the Beat groups and increasingly

TOM JONES IS SUPERB

†**"Green, Green Grass Of Home"/ "Promise Her Anything" (Decca).**
A GENTLY-SWAYING country flavoured rockaballad, with an easily hummable melody. A splendid, if subdued, performance by Tom—whose personality and individuality shine like a beacon.

Backing consists of organ, tinkling piano, choir and strings.

Sentimental, perhaps even if a bit square by Tom's standards, because it borders on the singalong. But it's extremely well done.

FLIP: A Bacharach-David number from the film of the same name. A sparkling finger-snapper, with Tom reverting to his familiar "It's Not Unusual" style.

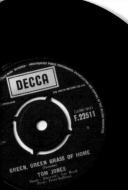

popular psychedelia and prog-rock bands. The year 1966 started out well for Jones, with the success of the theme tune from the fourth James Bond movie, *Thunderball*; this was soon followed by a Grammy for 'Best New Artist'.

'Green, Green Grass Of Home', which was based on a Jerry Lee Lewis original, achieved the notable feat of knocking the Beach Boys' epic 'Good Vibrations' off the UK No. 1 slot, and then went on to stay on top of the UK charts for a further seven weeks over the Christmas period (the album of the same name was a Top Five success).

In the '70s, Jones moved to America and became the highest-paid entertainer of the day, with a hugely successful TV show of his own and million-dollar residencies at a variety of Vegas casinos.

Jones fell out of favour with the record-buying public as the decade went on, but a return to form in the '80s saw him perform first with The Art Of Noise on a cover of Prince's 'Kiss', then enjoy his biggest-selling UK album with 2000's collaborative project *Reload*, featuring duets with Stereophonics' Kelly Jones among others.

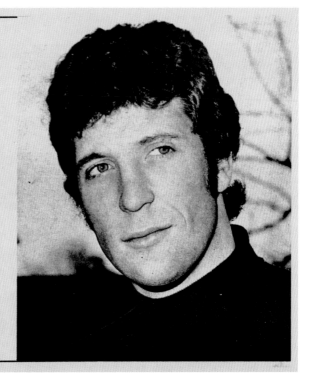

My sincere thanks to all NME readers for their votes and everyone who has helped to make 1966 such a successful year for me

TOM JONES

48 Come On Eileen
Dexy's Midnight Runners

Release Date: 3.07.82
No. Weeks In Chart: 17
Reached No. 1: 7.08.82
Total Sales: 1,201,000

This unique combination of Irish folk, searingly high-quality songwriting, inspired lyrics and unique imagery cemented Dexy's place in musical history.

After a tempestuous chart run of one previous No. 1, two Top 20 hits but three releases at No. 40 or below, British soul stylists Dexy's secured their place in musical history with this song. Named after an amphetamine used in northern soul circles, Dexy's Midnight Runners enjoyed unlikely but massive success with this masterpiece, which included horns, fiddles, banjos and tin whistles.

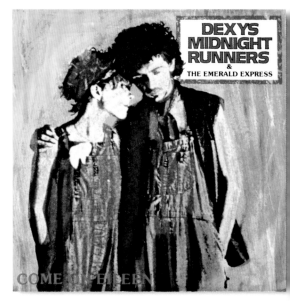

The exchange of the band's New York 'docker' look for a new 'gypsy chic' of dungarees and neckerchiefs met with considerable success. Seven months after 'Come On Eileen' topped the UK charts (1982's biggest seller), it repeated the position in the US.

Born in Wolverhampton to Irish parents, frontman Kevin Rowland's songwriting gift is widely recognised, but equally well known is the turbulent history behind the scenes. Rowland's disdain for the excesses of the music business fuelled endless sagas, personnel changes and arguments with record companies and the press. The band was dissolved in 1987, leaving a commercially unrewarding but nonetheless notorious solo career which saw Rowland take to festival stages in the late '90s wearing women's clothing . . . to scathing reviews. Dexy's Midnight Runners, however, remain one of the UK's finest bands of all time.

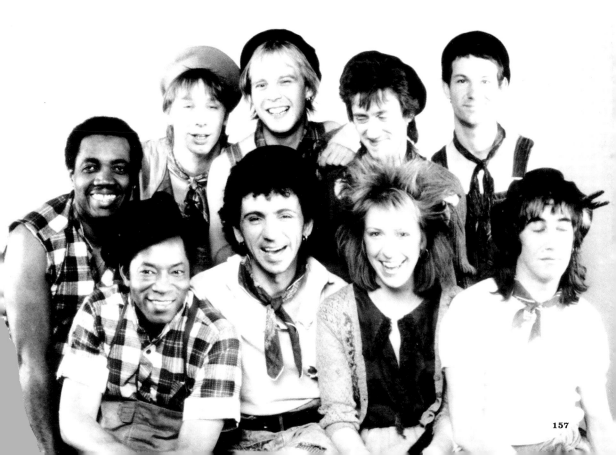

49 It Wasn't Me
Shaggy Featuring Rik Rok Ducent

Release Date: 10.03.01
No. Weeks In Chart: 20
Reached No. 1: 10.03.01
Total Sales: 1,180,708

This former US Marine and Gulf War veteran is a Grammy winner and the first reggae artist to perform in post-apartheid South Africa. His unique style – which he terms 'dog-a-muffin' – has seen him score a string of risqué, tongue-in-cheek UK Top Ten hits.

The world's foremost modern exponent of reggae, Jamaican-born Shaggy (Orville Burrell) has successfully taken that oft-maligned genre to the top of the world's charts. His unique bass vocals and heavy patois inflections had already earned him two previous No. 1s, with the reworking of the old Prince Buster classic, 'Oh Carolina', and 1995's 'Bombastic', which was set to the backdrop of Marvin Gaye's 'Let's Get It On'.

The tremendous advance hype for this single was sufficient to see it chart at No. 31 via import only. Three weeks later, the official release earned Shaggy a new entry at No. 1 and saw him score the year's biggest hit.

The single's enormous success helped to take his accompanying album, which carried the suitably modest title *Hot Shot*, to the No. 1 position all over the globe. Shaggy is famed for collaborating with a host of underground stars, and this best-selling single features the high-pitched super-melodious vocals of Rik Rok Ducent on the chorus.

Based on the theme of a so-called 'player' (West-Indian parlance for a male philanderer; the badge is meant to be worn with pride) who strenuously denies to his girlfriend that he has been unfaithful to her (despite eye-witnesses, video tapes and other irrefutable evidence), the song is typical of Shaggy's subject matter and self-proclaimed tongue-in-cheek comic attack.

The lyrics caused outrage in Shaggy's adoptive homeland of America, where the reference to 'banging on the bathroom floor' proved none too popular with the moral majority.

The publicity generated by the unashamed and overtly sexual lyrics was, however, somewhat more popular with Shaggy's record company – and the record-buying public.

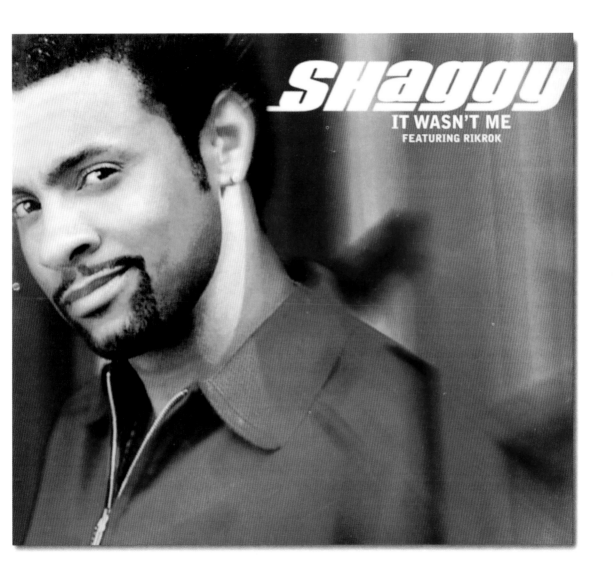

50 Heart Of Glass
Blondie

Release Date:	27.01.79
No. Weeks In Chart:	15
Reached No. 1:	3.02.79
Total Sales:	1,180,000

This cross-over disco hit, the band's most mainstream sound to date, enjoyed a month at the top spot.

'Heart of Glass' was Blondie's fifth UK Top 20 hit but only their first US No. 1. Europe and the UK had been the first to champion the refined punk-pop of New York's Blondie, led by the 'Monroe of the '70s', Deborah Harry. Harry initially experienced failure in the music scene of the late '60s with a hippie band called Wind In The Willows, followed by a pre-Blondie period which saw her working as a Playboy bunny girl and for the BBC in New York, among other jobs. During this time, legend has it that Debbie Harry declined a lift offered to her by the serial killer Ted Bundy.

Harry's productive creative partnership with Chris Stein and other members of Blondie made them one of the world's biggest acts at the turn of the '80s, and the commercial leaders of the so-called New Wave scene.

This disco-inflected hit single, the band's most mainstream sound to date, propelled the corresponding album, *Parallel Lines*, towards global sales of twenty million (their debut album *Blondie* was on Private Stock Records, home to David Soul – see No. 55). Interestingly, the first live incarnation of this track had been a more funk-oriented version.

The US finally bought into the Blondie phenomenon with 'Heart of Glass', the group's third single from their third album and a UK No. 1. The success of the single saw a party thrown by Andy Warhol at the famous New York Studio 54 nightclub. The band enjoyed three chart-toppers in their homeland to complement their rash of five in the UK.

The increasing emphasis placed on Debbie Harry's good looks and pin-up status, plus her solo career and movie ambitions, eventually led to the news of a split in October 1982. This was followed by a traumatic period spent nursing Stein, who had been her partner for some time, back from a critical illness.

Despite being originally and somewhat bizarrely criticised by some as 'emotionless', 'Heart of Glass' was remixed and re-entered at No. 16 in 1995, while a return to form in early 1999 saw a comeback single, 'Maria', earn them their sixth UK No. 1.

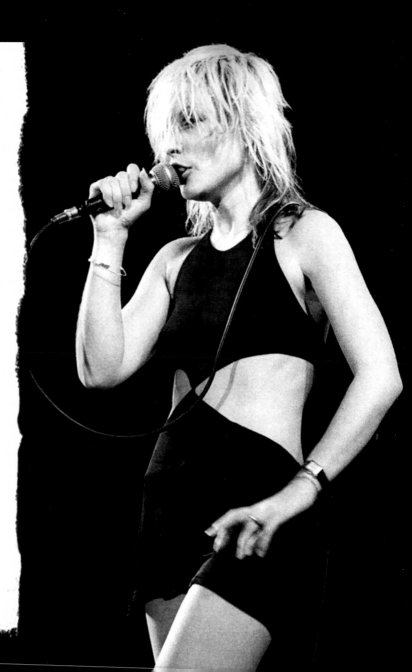

BLONDIE: Heart Of Glass (Chrysalis).

Hello, stranger. Look, we can't take back the things already said — but. . .well, I just had to let you know how much I love your "Heart Of Glass". It warmed the cockles of my kidneys, reminded me of just how great that first album was — maybe the finest debut vinyl of all time.

It made me think at long last of the girl striking kung fu poses at the Hammersmith Odeon in a black dress, dancing like a Tom Wolfe Peppermint Lounge Revisisted vision and effortlessly blowing Television out of West London. . .it made me think that *at long last* that girl was exactly where she should be today — down the disco (The Godmother of *Saturday Night Fever?* If you saw those first two UK dates in summer '77, you wouldn't raise an eyelash, kid), possessed by the soul of Donna Summer, the fire of Ronnie Spector and the spirit of Laura Nyro, knocking out the best dance-floor 45 of the week. Easy.

Which leaves Blondie: the Yellow Headed one torching it up like a black Julie London. I stand by all previous statements. I must doff my titfer to this.

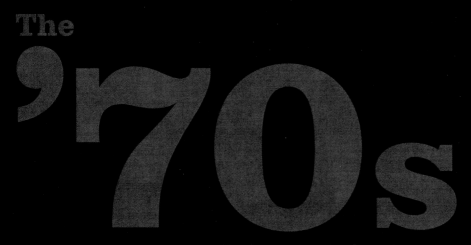

The '70s

The '70s were particularly notable for the ways in which the music scenes in the UK and the US diverged and journeyed in largely different directions.

After the demise of The Beatles, the US went for the heavier rock of Led Zeppelin as well as other stadium bands, such as Crosby, Stills and Nash and The Who. The UK, however, plumped for glam rock, with Bowie, Bolan, The Sweet and Slade leading the way. The decade started with the deaths of Jimi Hendrix, Janis Joplin and Jim Morrison. But from this bleak beginning grew some inspiring and, at times, revolutionary music.

Glam rock, arguably the ugliest genre in the history of music, also made its unforgettable mark on the decade's fashion. Belying their latter-day near-pantomime appearance, Slade were actually the first British skinhead band. After their image changed to one of spangly top hats and glam excess, the Wolverhampton band enjoyed six No. 1 hits (see No. 73). They even made their own feature film, *Slade In Flame* which, along with numerous TV appearances, showcased music's two most unlikely heroes – the mightily sideburned Noddy Holder and the horizontally fringed Dave Hill.

Disco was also a massive '70s craze. The box-office smash *Saturday Night Fever* was the obvious commercial highpoint, paving the way

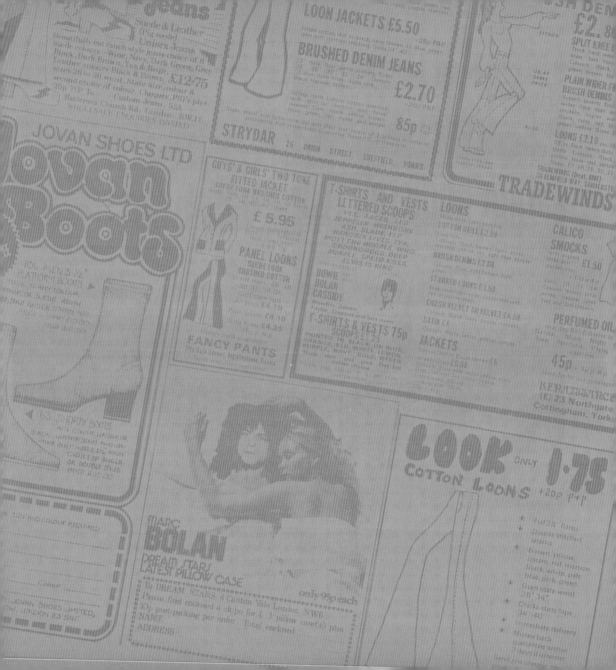

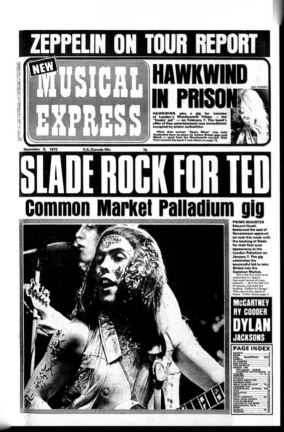

ZEPPELIN ON TOUR REPORT

NEW **MUSICAL EXPRESS**

HAWKWIND IN PRISON

HAWKWIND play a gig for inmates of London's Wandsworth Prison — the "freaks jail" on February 7. The band's offer of free entertainment was immediately accepted by prison authorities.

When their current 'Space Ritual' tour ends Hawkwind have no plans for further British gigs until March — apart from the Wandsworth concert. Nick Kent reviews the band's new album on page 12.

December 9, 1972   U.S./Canada 90c.   7p.

SLADE ROCK FOR TED
Common Market Palladium gig

PRIME MINISTER Edward Heath bestowed the seal of Government approval on rock this week with the booking of Slade for their first-ever appearance at the London Palladium on January 7. The gig celebrates the successful bid to take Britain into the Common Market.

This is the first event to be announced in a special free-week festival of major concerts — all in the first half of January and staged under the heading 'Fanfare for Europe.' They cover every aspect of music. Further details page 3.

McCARTNEY RY COODER DYLAN JACKSONS

PAGE INDEX

for acts such as Boney M to reap huge sales from the pockets of a nation of wide-collared fashion disasters (see No.'s 5, 10).

However, the most obvious stylistic legacy of the '70s is punk. This most incendiary of beasts single-handedly redefined popular culture. The musical environment into which gate-crashed this firebrand was a tepid and bloated world of over-priced stadium gigs and mammoth world tours. The only real grass-roots alternative was

the pub-rock scene, or perhaps a few snippets from the blossoming New York scene. Led Zeppelin, David Bowie, Yes and Pink Floyd had taken pop-star status onto a level far removed from their fans, composing for instruments that cost small fortunes; playing with calculated virtuosity in 64-track studios.

The Sex Pistols were the nucleus; but once they had sworn on Bill Grundy's television show, the floodgates were opened. Musically there was little to tempt Britain's youth away from the wave of snarling punk venom. The Eagles had become the first group to achieve platinum status with their *Greatest Hits 1971–75* album, while the Bay City Rollers, Elton John and Kiki Dee dominated the charts of the mid-'70s, along with the likes of Brotherhood of Man and Showaddywaddy (see No. 84). Such fare was the fuel to punk's fire.

Punks quickly established their own identity. Individuality was the key, with hand-sprayed clothes, ripped trousers and extravagant hairstyles. In London, many of the key players were clothed by Malcolm McLaren and Vivienne Westwood's seminal 'Sex' shop, decking out Johnny Rotten in his infamous 'bondage' trousers. These became staple items of punk's stereotypical look, and were first sold as early as September 1976 as a direct offshoot of the more fetish-based clothing the couple usually offered. In the provinces, improvisation resulted in crudely painted T-shirts, mohair jumpers and tight trousers. One interesting feature was the occasional trend to misappropriate elements of teddy-boy fashion, such as the string tie that Rotten and McLaren were often seen sporting, drainpipe trousers, or Sid's drape jacket – all of these items were worn, much to the annoyance of the purist teds. Ironically, the chart impact of the leading punk bands was somewhat limited, and none appear in this list. Yet their social and cultural impact has resounded down the years.

The decade closed with the grim urban reality of Coventry's Two Tone scene, featuring bands such as The Specials and north London's Madness. The sartorial origins of the scene were embedded deep in Jamaica with the rude-boy culture of the late '50s. Rude boys took great pride in their attire – extremely neat suits were made by backstreet tailors with noticeably short trousers, usually in two-tone fabrics. The outfits were completed with loafers and optional pork-pie hats, sometimes called 'stingy brims' or 'bluebeat hats'.

The first UK rude boys wore loafers – usually black – and their shirts and hats were often far more colourful than the later monochrome style. This was a direct descendant of the extravagant tailoring of the Jamaicans, although the style would, predictably, be toned down for the British public. Rude girl fashion often consisted of tight, knee-length skirts, often with zipper sides, sleeveless shirts, frequently in black and white, with dark red lipstick and shoulder-length hair.

Meanwhile, across the Atlantic, the underground development of a fledgling hip-hop and rap scene was beginning to make its presence felt – in time, this would become the most refreshing and innovative new genre to be introduced to the music scene in years.

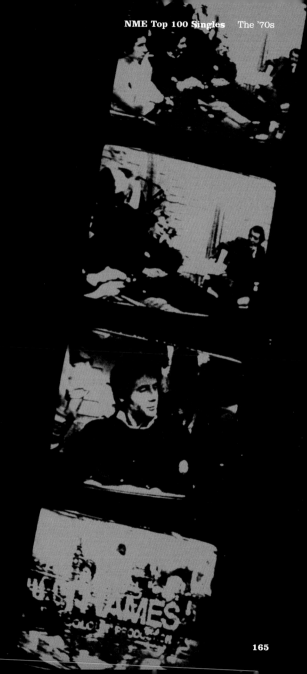

51 Mary's Boy Child
Harry Belafonte

Release Date: 1.11.57
No. Weeks In Chart: 19
Reached No. 1: 22.11.57
Total Sales: 1,175,000

This is the only song to be included in this list twice, although this hit single was not actually Belafonte's most famous song – that accolade goes to '(Day-O) The Banana Boat Song'.

This seven-week Christmas No. 1 (see also No. 10) was the biggest-selling single for Belafonte, an actor-turned-singer-turned-civil rights campaigner and political activist. A career on Broadway – a thing almost unheard of for a black man at that time – was shunned after Belafonte tired of the curfews and racial segregation. So instead, he opened up his own hamburger joint, The Sage, in Greenwich Village, New York.

There, Belafonte would sing after-hours to both customers and friends, drawing heavily on his love of West Indian calypso music – a passion dating from his pre-World War II years in Jamaica. This genre was to provide him with his commercial breakthrough.

As the so-called 'King of Calypso', Harry Belafonte was to enjoy several years as the top-earning black entertainer in the world, at one point being paid the then staggering sum of $1 million for a residency at a top hotel. His *Calypso* album of 1955 topped the US charts for 31 weeks, leading some observers to suggest that this genre would soon replace the 'fad' of rock 'n' roll. (Ironically, this song was toppled from the UK's No. 1 spot by Jerry Lee Lewis' 'Great Balls of Fire'.) Belafonte also starred in eight feature films during his musical heyday.

During the '70s and onwards, he increasingly turned away from music and towards civil rights and politics. He was a prime mover behind 'USA for Africa', the 1985 American answer to Bob Geldof's Band Aid, and has since become a Unicef Goodwill Ambassador as well as a constantly active and deeply respected campaigner on various issues.

Interestingly, for his 1961 *Midnight Special* record, he paid a local harmonica player by the name of Bob Dylan $50 to play on a session (Dylan is credited as 'Blind Boy Grunt').

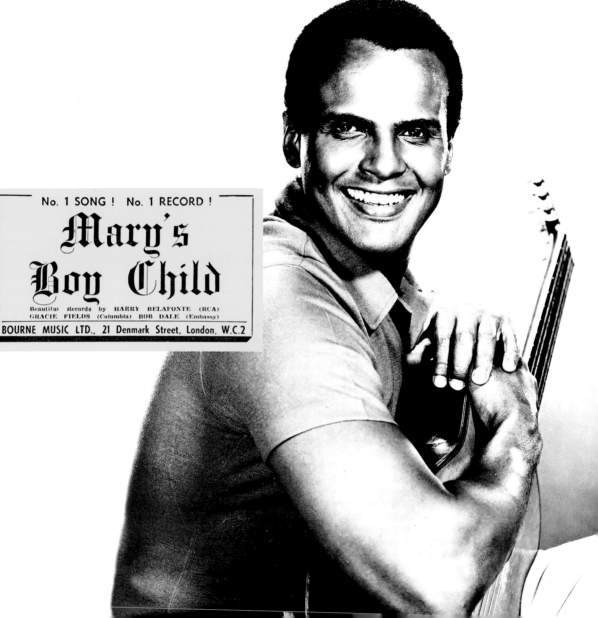

No. 1 SONG !   No. 1 RECORD !

Mary's Boy Child

Beautiful Records by HARRY BELAFONTE (RCA)
GRACIE FIELDS (Columbia) BOB DALE (Embassy)

BOURNE MUSIC LTD., 21 Denmark Street, London, W.C.2

52

The Last Waltz
Engelbert Humperdinck

Release Date:	23.08.67
No. Weeks In Chart:	27
Reached No. 1:	6.09.67
Total Sales:	1,160,000

Known to some fans as 'The Humpster', Humperdinck can boast the largest fan club in the world with eight million members and a staggering total of over 130 million records sold worldwide.

After the debut No. 1 of his single 'Release Me' (see No. 35), Humperdinck quickly became a globally successful vocalist. As the British press announced that the Beat invasion of America was fading fast, Humperdinck and his stablemate Tom Jones chiselled out a healthy niche appealing to a more mature demograph. Jones' hip-swivelling pop raunch formed a neat contrast to Humperdinck's mellower lounge-king approach, often sourced from the country genre, which suited his silken voice perfectly.

With 'Release Me' still in the charts six months after its release, 'The Last Waltz' gave Engelbert his second biggest hit single ever. A total of nine Top 20 hits between 1967 and 1970 helped make him a staple of the newly broadcasting Adult Contemporary Radio.

The song was eventually replaced at the top by the Bee Gees' first No. 1, '(The Night The Lights Went Out In) Massachusetts'.

Engelbert's success continued into the early '70s, when he was often the UK's best-selling artist. His career has recently enjoyed an Indian summer, due to his rediscovery by a new generation of lounge-music lovers who enjoy his famous easy-listening classics, along with those of other masters of the genre, such as Burt Bacharach and Tony Bennett. And he is still touring; his act these days includes impressions of Elvis, Julio Iglesias and Dean Martin as well as those much-loved ballads.

His impact is not restricted merely to the music scene. Modern fashion historians have noted that Engelbert wore outrageous leather jumpsuits and sideburns long before Elvis (the two were close friends).

Among his other achievements is the theme song to the Beavis and Butthead movie, entitled 'Lesbian Seagull'.

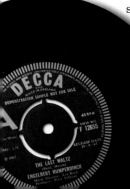

DON'T CALL ME ENGELBERT

ENGELBERT HUMPERDINCK, looking rather like a Mississippi gambler in immaculate grey suit and waistcoat, puffed thoughtfully on his cigar. "The next step for me now is to break into films," he said, blowing out a cloud of smoke. "I've already had about six offers—one of them from Hollywood to star with Steve McQueen. But until the exact contract we want comes along we'll just wait."

Engel, as he now wants to be called, was in his dressing room at the BBC's Playhouse Theatre waiting to do his spot on the "Joe Loss Pop Show."

The voice of the compere Tony Hall suddenly came over the speaker " . . . . and this week's special guest Engelbert Humperdinck ! "

The audience burst into thunderous applause and the Joe Loss Orchestra struck up its opening theme.

Praise and adulation are things which Engel has come

NMExclusive
by NORRIE DRUMMOND

to expect wherever he goes nowadays. He recently played a ballroom date where he had the shirt ripped off his back.

"Half of the audience were youngsters and they all stood at the front," he said, " but behind them were a lot of much older women. Some of them fifty and over."

This, I'm sure, is one of the qualities which will keep Engel at the top for a long time. He appeals not only to teenage record-buyers but to older audiences as well.

He can play in clubs or ballrooms and he will probably star at London's famous " Talk Of The Town " just as soon as a date can be fixed. Offers keep pouring in from continental countries and now America—where " Release Me " is at No. 4—wants him too.

"I'd like to go out to America in a few weeks' time," he said.

"I want to see what the scene's like over there. But we'll probably wait and see how the next record issued there does before we make any definite plans.

(*These were finalised late Tuesday night and he flies out next Monday, returning the following Friday. See full details on centre pages.—*EDITOR.)

"I don't think 'There Goes My Everything' will be the follow-up in America. We've still to decide what it will be."

Quick success

Engelbert Humperdinck's success has happened so quickly and become so widespread that one could be forgiven for thinking that he must have changed.

Certainly he can now afford to do most of the things he wants

He can buy the best suits, the best cars, the best cigars. But apart from his Jaguar and some new clothes for him and his family he has bought little else.

He still lives in the same flat in Hammersmith with his wife and children.

"Apart from new carpets our flat is exactly the same as it was 18 months ago. Naturally we'll move to a new house sometime but just when I don't know."

Engelbert estimates that 12-18 months ago his annual income was somewhere in the region of £500 a year. "We really were having a rough time," he said.

"Then came the Song Contest in Knokke last year. Fortunately we won and with the prize money I raced home to pay the rent. We were almost on the point of being thrown out."

Then, of course, work came a lot more frequently until now when he really is a great

is able to pick and choose the job he wants.

"Security is a wonderful feeling," said Engelbert happily. " Knowing that people want you and not having to scrape around picking up the odd job here and there."

Engelbert, looking bronzed after a recent holiday in Portugal—the first he's been able to afford for a long time—smiled contentedly. " Yes, really is a great f

SO SQUARE, ENGELBERT!

*"The Last Waltz"/"That Promise" (Decca).

OOZING with saccharine, dripping with corn and bursting with sentiment, this is bound to be another smash for Engelbert. It's more than square, it's cube—but it's loaded with sing-along appeal and nostalgia.

The rhythm is blatantly an old-fashioned waltz—lilting and swaying maybe, but hardly the stuff for mod dancers.

The verses aren't particularly inspiring, but the disc really comes alive in the four-times-repeated chorus, which is very catchy and features a vocal group lustily joining in with the soloist.

And in case you don't know the words, there's a la-la chorus you can hum along with!

FLIP: This gives Hump an opportunity to display his ability as a dynamic and sophisticated performer. A vibrantly-handled jog-trotter with brass-and-strings backing.

53 Bright Eyes
Art Garfunkel

Release Date: 3.03.79
No. Weeks In Chart: 19
Reached No. 1: 14.04.79
Total Sales: 1,155,000

The film about a group of rabbits looking for a safe haven gave Art some welcome chart success.

After Simon & Garfunkel split in 1970, Art spent some time acting (*Catch 22* and *Carnal Knowledge*) before turning to a solo career in 1973 with the indicative soft melodies of his beautiful counter-tenor voice on *Angel Clare*. 'Bright Eyes' was his second UK No. 1 after the hit album *Breakaway* produced the single 'I Only Have Eyes For You'.

This song was taken from the soundtrack of the enormously successful movie, *Watership Down* – an animated adaptation of Richard Adams' 1972 novel – directed by Martin Rosen and including the voices of John Hurt and Richard Briers. Its cinematic success gave Art some welcome chart success, coming after a period in which his records had struggled to match the rich pickings of Simon & Garfunkel's fertile phase in the mid-'60s. Like this single, his 1979 album *Scissors Cut* failed to make the Top 100 in the US. By contrast, this song spent six weeks at the top of the UK list.

The following year, a Simon & Garfunkel reunion gig in Central Park attracted over 500,000 people. However, the subsequent international tour was followed by another split for the duo, who were originally called Tom &

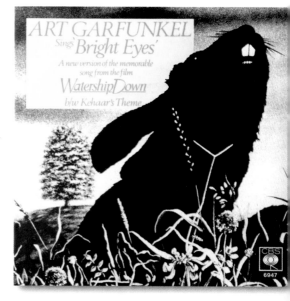

Jerry. In the mid-'80s, Garfunkel took to long-distance walking, his treks including a month-long trawl across Japan and annual walks across the US, during which he would write poetry. Garfunkel is one of the charts' more intellectual artists, possessing a degree in Art History and a Masters in Mathematics.

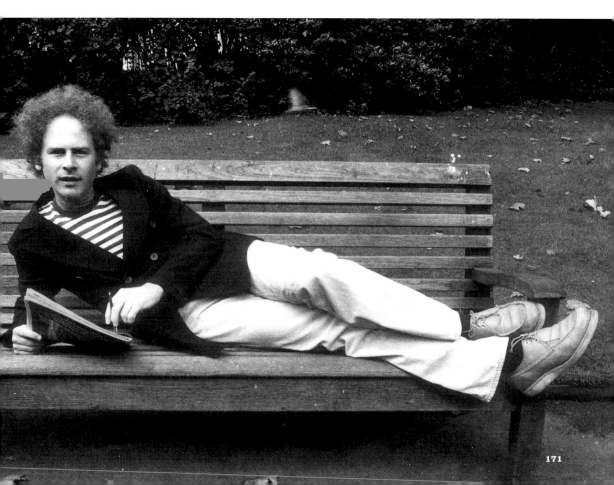

54 Heartbeat/Tragedy
Steps

Release Date: 21.11.98
No. Weeks In Chart: 30
Reached No. 1: 9.01.99
Total Sales: 1,150,285

Their thirteen consecutive Top Five singles constitute an achievement only bettered by The Beatles.

In the space of five years, Steps enjoyed fifteen Top 20 singles, and in 1999 they performed on the biggest pop tour to date in UK history. This was their first No. 1, a double A-side of a slow ballad and a Bee Gees cover – the Christmas party popularity of 'Tragedy' fuelled heavy sales of this, their fourth single, which took it to the top spot more than two months after it had been released, something of an unusual feat in a chart era characterised by straight-to-No. 1 new entries.

The band's easy-to-follow dance routines and cheeky image proved a massive smash with younger audiences, who flocked in their droves to buy their records. Ironically, their chart debut was perhaps their weakest song, the potential one-hit wonder of the line-dancing novelty hit, '5-6-7-8'. The single has the 'honour' of being the biggest-selling song of the '90s not to reach the Top Ten.

After this uncertain start, the group quickly garnered a reputation for both hi-energy covers and pop-classic originals. Their No. 1 second album, *Steptacular*, went on to become one of the biggest-selling of the decade, shifting

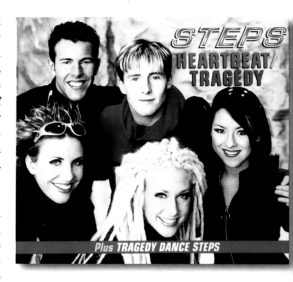

nearly two million units and winning the group their own TV show in the process. Steps subsequently spoiled thousands of pre-teen (and gay men's) Yuletides by announcing their split on Boxing Day 2001.

At that point, they could boast total sales of twelve million records and sell-outs of over 120 arenas. Surprisingly, their only other chart-topper was 2000's 'Stomp'.

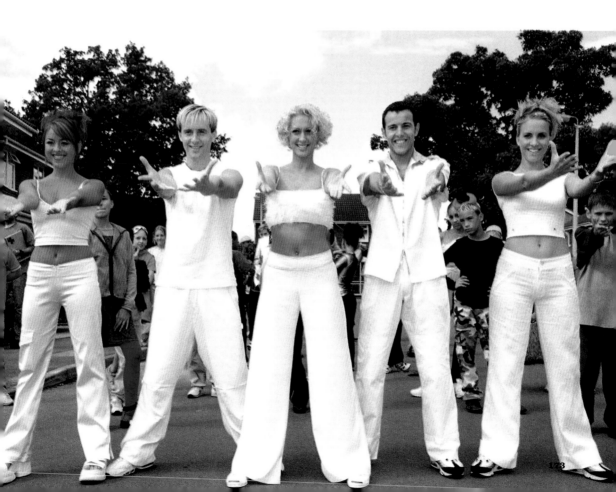

55 Don't Give Up On Us
David Soul

Release Date:	18.12.76
No. Weeks In Chart:	16
Reached No. 1:	15.01.77
Total Sales:	1,145,000

This Tony Macauley-penned smash hit single, pleading for a love not to die, saw Soul become Britain's premier heart-throb, with a look that appealed to all ages.

An American of Norwegian descent and the son of a Lutheran minister and professor, David Solberg spent much of his childhood in desolate post-war East Germany. Turning down the offer of a pro-baseball contract to study political science in Mexico, Solberg subsequently pursued a music career, playing for $5 a night in bars and supporting himself by working as a truck driver, bank clerk and selling encyclopedias door to door.

His reputation as a folk singer blossomed, aided by the curious gimmick of wearing a ski mask. However, it was his acting ability, through various theatre and TV roles (as David Soul) that won him global fame – his lead part in the smash '70s police TV series *Starsky and Hutch* has made an indelible mark on popular culture.

The success of this single saw Soul become Britain's premier heart-throb, earning him five Top 20 hits at a time when punk was ravaging the UK. At one point, he talked a female fan out of suicide in the north of England, after desperate UK police had called him at his Los Angeles home.

DAVID SOUL: Don't Give Up On Us (Private Stock). One of the TV cops' answer to the Odd Couple. It looks as though, with his album charting at 20, David Soul can win over the hearts and the wallets of millions even when not holding his partner's hand. Balladeering strings and don't give up on us, baby. Actually he hasn't got a bad voice. But would you trust Lassky or Crutch to search your kid brother?

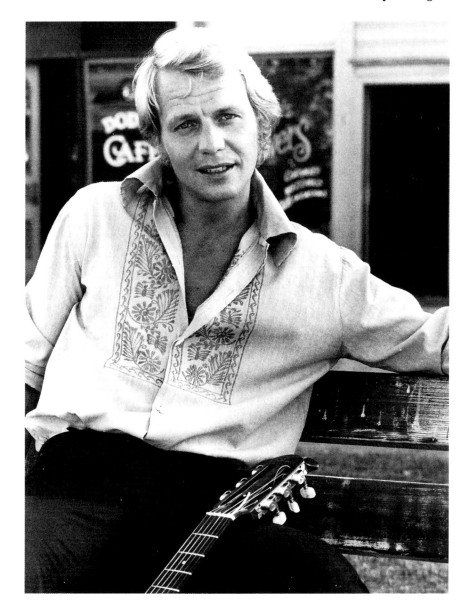

Festivals

> I regarded the whole thing as a cross
> between a harvest festival and a pop festival.

Michael Eavis, Glastonbury Organiser

Many see the Monterey Pop Festival as the first of the great rock festivals. Descended from the Monterey Jazz and Folk Festival, this 1967 event saw a spectacularly destructive performance by The Who and, into the bargain, Jimi Hendrix's infamous guitar-burning extravaganza during his extraordinary rendition of 'Wild Thing'.

Since then a whole crop of festivals has evolved – Woodstock, Live Aid, Glastonbury, Reading and Lollapalooza, to name but a few. British festivals are led by the Glastonbury weekend, attended most years by tens of thousands prepared to face the usual onslaught of mud baths and long toilet queues. Despite this, the weekend has a cherished place in the hearts of most British festival-goers.

Its enigmatic organiser, farmer Michael, revealed how this legendary festival started off in bizarre circumstances. 'The first problem was that I knew nothing about the music business. I started by ringing up Colston Hall in Bristol to ask how I could get in touch with pop groups. A chap there gave me the name of an agent, and the agent put me in touch with the Kinks, who agreed to appear for £500, which

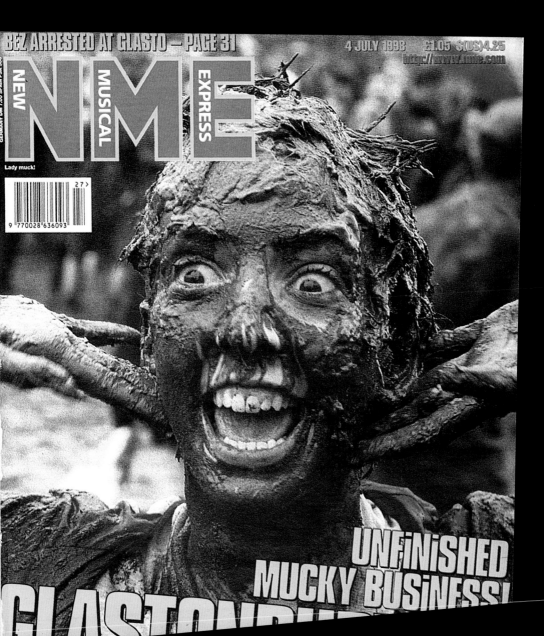

BEZ ARRESTED AT GLASTO – PAGE 31

4 JULY 1998   £1.05 $(US)4.25
http://www.nme.com

NEW

NME

MUSICAL

EXPRESS

Lady muck!

27>

9 770028 636093

UNFiNiSHED
MUCKY BUSINESS!

GLASTONBURY

was a lot of money for me to pull out of a milk churn . . . I was ready to give up. I woke up every morning before milking time worrying about how much it was costing me, thinking it was doomed to failure . . . '

At that first Glastonbury festival, back in September 1970, Eavis handed out free milk and provided a large ox roast (which was hijacked by hungry Hells Angels). Despite local pubs posting signs saying 'Hippies Keep Out', there was a strong turnout. However, Eavis still managed to lose £1,500. Through the more hippified days of the '70s, Glastonbury survived and continued to grow, eventually seeing massive headline slots by global acts such as Prodigy, Pulp, Radiohead and New Order (see No. 76). Today, Glastonbury perhaps qualifies as the definitive UK festival.

Nonetheless, pivotal Reading performances, such as Nirvana's last-ever UK show in 1992 amid rumours of Cobain returning to heroin use and a possible no-show, have kept that August Bank Holiday weekender high on the list of festival-goers' priorities.

Glastonbury's problems with overcrowding in the late '90s were dwarfed by much earlier outdoor extravaganzas. The famous 'loved-up' Woodstock festival of August 1969 was intended to be a highly organised and commercially minded event.

Originally, 186,000 tickets were sold, with police expecting around 200,000 people to attend. However, on the weekend in question, over one million people turned up at Max Yasgur's farm in Bethel, New York. Within hours, the $18 entrance fee had been

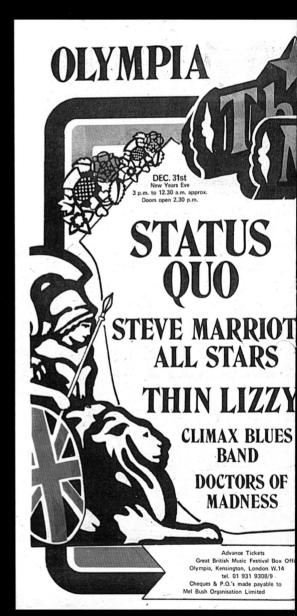

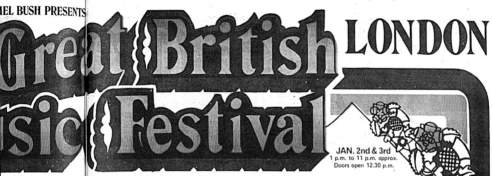

MEL BUSH PRESENTS

Great British Music Festival

LONDON

JAN. 2nd & 3rd
1 p.m. to 11 p.m. approx.
Doors open 12.30 p.m.

1 p.m. to 11 p.m. approx. JAN 1st Doors open 12.30 p.m.

PROCOL HARUM

BARCLAY JAMES HARVEST

BAKER GURVITZ ARMY

JACK THE LAD

JOHN MILES

SNAFU

BAD COMPANY
NAZARETH
RONNIE LANE'S SLIM CHANCE
PRETTY THINGS
BE·BOP DELUXE
CHARLIE

Agents
All branches Virgin Records tel. 01/727 8070
London Theatre Bookings tel. 01/439 3371
Hime & Addison Manchester tel. 061/834 8019
Glasgow Apollo tel. 041/332 6055
All Box Offices open Sat. 22 Nov. 10 a.m.

TICKETS £3.50 EACH DAY
No reserved seating

Peter Grainey Graphics, Bournemouth

abandoned and the event turned into a free festival, as security could do little to keep the swarming masses at bay. As the most chronicled example of its genre, these 'Three Days of Peace And Music' also saw three deaths, two births and four miscarriages. Elsewhere, other open-air shows have become bywords for events often totally unrelated to music – the fatal stabbing at The Rolling Stones' Altamont show in 1969 is a case in point.

As the years went by, festivals mutated into a more potent force. Instead of being a gathering for gathering's sake, the mass events were turned to political or social ends. Anti-racism, gay liberation, animal rights, the homeless and scores of charitable and other issues have benefited from festival income over the years. The biggest fundraiser of them all, of course, was 1985's Live Aid.

The brainchild of Bob Geldof, lead singer of the Boomtown Rats – who had been prompted to act by a shocking BBC documentary about the Ethiopian famine – the event followed on from Geldof's collaborative Christmas single, 'Do They Know It's Christmas?' This featured a host of British names and became the second best-selling UK single of all time (see No. 2). By the end of the day, with a simultaneous event in Philadelphia's JFK Stadium, and watched by a global audience of over 1.5 billion people, Geldof and his colleagues had started a phenomenon that would go on to generate over $70 million for aid relief.

Lollapalooza re-invented the festival for the modern era with a myriad of musical styles accompanied by information about a variety of

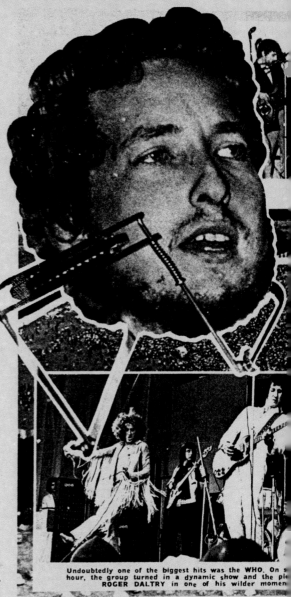

Undoubtedly one of the biggest hits was the WHO. On s hour, the group turned in a dynamic show and the pie ROGER DALTRY in one of his wilder momen

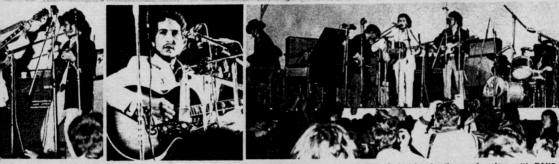

...e three-day event, **BOB DYLAN** in a rare festival picture close-up (left) is almost hidden behind a jungle of mikes as he plays with **BAND** ... **DANKO** and **ROBBIE ROBERTSON**. His shortened act gave rise to a row but most people were happy with what they saw of the legendary ... the far right, pianist **RICHARD MANUEL**, organist **GARTH HUDSON** and drummer **LEVON HELM** can also be seen.

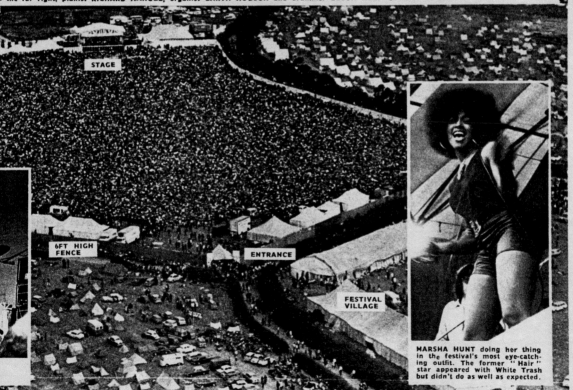

STAGE

6FT HIGH FENCE

ENTRANCE

FESTIVAL VILLAGE

MARSHA HUNT doing her thing in the festival's most eye-catching outfit. The former " Hair " star appeared with White Trash but didn't do as well as expected.

'hot' issues. Each stadium-sized show had stalls organised by major and minor protest groups, such as Greenpeace, gun-control lobbyists and civil liberties groups. Tattooists and fire-eaters added to the general bohemian atmosphere, and the resultant tour package was a phenomenal success – in many respects, this was the true Woodstock 2. (The real Woodstock 2, in 1994, was generally viewed as deeply disappointing and having been hijacked by corporate money-men.) More recently, the Beastie Boys' Tibetan Freedom concerts have also captured youth's imagination, despite being struck by lightning (during the 1998 show).

Festivals offer smaller bands a unique opportunity to play in front of gargantuan crowds – few acts can fill Shea Stadium with 56,000 screaming fans (see The Beatles, No.'s 8, 14, 20, 27 and 32) or swell the area around the Berlin Wall with 400,000 (see No. 78). Yet, paradoxically, festivals are often the perfect venue for more mainstream artists to play to thousands of more alternative-minded music lovers: Tom Jones (see No. 47) has played on the main stages of numerous UK festivals. Even acts such as Boney M still headline more local events, such as the 2002 Clare Festival in Suffolk, a quarter of a century after their chart heyday (see No.'s 5 and 10).

Leaving aside the festival saturation of the late '90s, which saw several high-profile cancellations, the experience of a weekend with a tent, a few mates and a field shared with 50,000 strangers remains one of those rites of passage which – weather permitting – will, hopefully, always be with us.

200,000

FOUR days before he was due to appear at the Is
Dylan told me that the more he played the be
view of that, that the should perform for only just ove
was: " I was here at five-thirty, ready to go on, b
played long enough, I didn't want to go on much lon

There was definitely a severe mix-up about the time Dylan and the Band should have gone on stage. Journalists were originally told nine pm until midnight, but this was altered during the afternoon. In the evening, approaching seven, it was changed again, but co-promoter Ron Faulk wasn't able to give a definite time.

But Dyl sink Is reports

When Dylan eventually appeared, dressed in a white suit, smiling broadly and being handed his guitar by an assistant, the crowd of almost two hundred thousand (rather less than had been expected), gave him a mighty roar of approval. At least they hadn't minded the wait.

Watched by a celebrity-packed audience which included John Lennon, George Harrison, Ringo Starr, Keith Richard, Bill Wyman, Charlie Watts, Steve Winwood, Jim Capaldi, Francoise Hardy, Amen Corner's Alan Jones and Mike Smith, actress Jane Fonda and her husband Roger Vadim, and actor Richard Johnson. Dylan opened with " Every-

thing She Needs " which
about the shortest thing he
He hunched his shoulders
as he went into " Mr. Tar
Man " and " Maggie's Farn
the atmosphere was getting
The Band, who hadn't been
in their own spot, sound
behind Dylan — the two ac
together really well.

All his numbers were fami
as promised, new arrangem
been worked out specially
festival " Lay Lady Lay " g
round of applause as it bega
such things can be jud
audience response, looks like

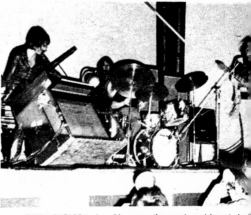

KEITH EMERSON gives his organ the usual punishment dur
NICE's show-stopping act. **BLINKY DAVIDSON** is half-hidden
his cymbals and **LEE JACKSON** watched Keith for musica

r approval

Including John, George Ringo and wives!

...estival on Sunday, Bob
...ed all the stranger, in
... explanation afterwards
... waiting until eleven. I

In't quite
Wight,
rd Green

...gle.
... we heard "Immigrants," the
...ic "Like A Rolling Stone"
... I'll Be Your Baby Tonight."
...me, "Let's Go Get Stoned"
...bout the highspot and it was
...ointing when, just after mid-
...Dylan walked off stage.
... crowd obviously expected
...but they didn't get it. It was
... and several people gathered
...age to protest about the
...ess of Dylan's act. Despite that
...nqualified success.
...Band's set was as nice as
... expected, the sound was good
...re wasn't the originality we

hoped for. The piano played a heavy
part in a spot that consisted mainly
of numbers from the "Big Pink"
album. Of the selections, "The
Weight" and the Four Tops'
"Loving You" were about the best
and most well-received.

For the rest of the three-day event,
Friday night was the night of the
Nice. There is no other conceivable
way to describe what I regard to be
one of their best sets yet.

Of course, there was an encore
and it had to be "America," but it
proved to be an encore and a half
— almost a show in itself.

We saw Keith Emerson standing on
the organ and playing at the same
time, no mean feat, Brian Davison in
really great form on drums and Lee
Jackson doing good things with his
bass. "Karelia" was as interesting
as ever and Tchaikovsky's "Path-
etique" (with a little doctoring) was
a fine starter.

The one piece that really scored
for me was Tim Hardin's "Hang On
To A Dream" which is on the new
album. Keith ran up and down the
scales on his piano while Lee
injected into the song a soft quality I
didn't know he possessed. It got all
very jazzy and swung like the Young
Holt Trio. Ten out of ten, me lads.

The Bonzo Dog Band preceded the
Nice and, as usual, relied heavily
upon visual humour for appeal.

Bobby Pickett's "Monster Mash"
was treated well and "Ventricles Of
Your Mind" and "Urban Space-

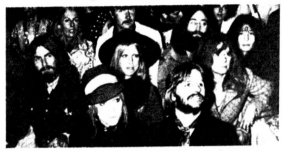

Three BEATLES — GEORGE, JOHN and RINGO — with their respective wives attended the star-packed festival to watch DYLAN on the
final night. Here they are seated in the special private enclosure.

man" were received enthusiastical-
ly.

After all the ballyhoo and balloney
about Marsha Hunt I expected great
things. But I really must admit
disappointment. After the show, she
told me: "It was a drag." And
that's just about it.

Wearing black leather shorts, boots
and gloves she gyrated about the
stage in what was, presumably,
meant to be an erotic manner. Sorry,
love, it left me cold.

For the record, her numbers

included "Wild Thing," "Walk On
Gilded Splinters" and "My World Is
Empty Without You." Oh well,
perhaps it will be better next time.

During all the goings-on, I met
Noel Redding who was as staggering
as ever. He said: "We couldn't get
the Rolls on the ferry," and left it at
that.

Later, he spent a long time
chatting to Jane Fonda and Roger
Vadim and they agreed that he could
send them a film story and music he
has written!

Moody Blue Ray Thomas cadged a
fag off me and promised good things
to come. Which they did.

Strong point

The ever-popular "Dr. Living-
stone" from "In Search Of The Lost
Chord" sounded as good on stage as
it does on record — this is one of the
strong points about the Moodies,
their ability to reproduce almost
exactly their recorded sound on
"live" appearances. If only a few
more groups would please copy.

Justin Hayward and Ray Thomas
sang "Never Comes The Day"
together and we heard "Peak
Hour" and "Tuesday Afternoon"
which was a hit in America but not
a single here. "Nights In White
Satin" was very popular with the
crowd who dug every minute of the
group's act.

Loud and prolonged cheers and
cries for more brought the boys back
for "Ride My See Saw," a pleasant
little rock and roll number. I think
what people liked most was the
Moodies' professionalism and musi-
c'anship. And that is a good thing.

The Who made their usual spectacular entrance — this time by
helicopter. All of us backstage got
covered in all sorts of flying muck

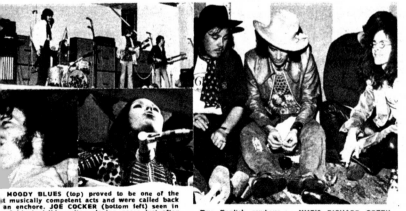

MOODY BLUES (top) proved to be one of the
...t musically competent acts and were called back
...an enchore. JOE COCKER (bottom left) seen in
... of his invisible guitar playing poses just after
...long U.S. visit. JULIE FELIX (bottom right)
... a popular hit on Sunday afternoon, getting
tremendous applaiuse for her warm act.

Two English cowboys — NME'S RICHARD GREEN
(left) and FAT MATTRESS lead singer NEIL LANDON
discuss tobacco merits while NOEL REDDING finds
the whole thing a big laugh.

Continued on page 14

56 I Love You Love Me Love
Gary Glitter

Release Date: 17.11.73
No. Weeks In Chart: 14
Reached No. 1: 17.11.73
Total Sales: 1,140,000

Nothing if not persistent, the now out of favour Gary Glitter was yet another alter ego of rock veteran Paul Gadd, breaking onto the scene after twelve years in the wilderness.

Such is the notoriety generated by his latter-day convictions on child pornography charges that it is easy to forget Glitter's sizeable chart success.

Nothing if not persistent, Gary Glitter was yet another alter ego of rock veteran Paul Gadd (Vicky Vomit and Stanley Sparkle were also mooted). This new persona was launched by 'burying' the records and memorabilia of his previous incarnation, Paul Raven, in a coffin on the River Thames.

Glitter's origins in a late '50s skiffle group were a long way from the eventual chart-topping, platform-heeled silver-foil caricature that this single – which went straight in at No. 1 and stayed there for a month – represented.

The record's chanting and anthemic vocals were worked to good effect and championed notably by BBC Radio One. It was a lucrative formula, and one that enabled Gadd to spend extravagantly – and curiously. At one point he laid out £6,000 just on motorised curtains!

Gadd, a former warm-up man for *Ready, Steady, Go!*, enjoyed eleven consecutive Top Ten hits between 1972 and 1975 (in total he enjoyed twelve Top Ten hits; this last one did not come until 1984) and three Top Ten albums under the name of Gary Glitter. But after glam rock faded, his life fell apart: bankruptcy, tax debts, retirements and comebacks, personal problems and an overdose of sleeping pills dominated his days.

A return to favour in the '80s saw Gary Glitter support Wham! at their farewell Wembley gig in 1986, before playing popular arena-filling annual Christmas tours. But then came his dramatic fall from grace. He now spends his wigless days travelling covertly around the globe hounded by paparazzi.

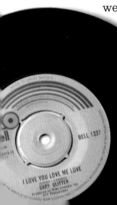

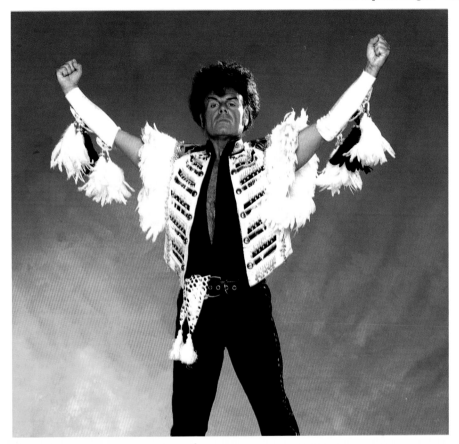

GARY GLITTER: "I Love You Love Me Love" (Bell). *I think great it's pretty all good right. El Glittroid manifests himself once more with a thoroughly reprehensible record with an unsettling resemblance to a drunken working men's club singing a fifties' doo-wop ballad. My informants tell me that Gary is going to use this song to strip to on stage, which should result in the most horrifying piece of over-exposure since Watergate. Talking of which, see Charlie Drake review.*

57 Tainted Love
Soft Cell

Release Date: 1.08.81
No. Weeks In Chart: 44
Reached No. 1: 5.09.81
Total Sales: 1,135,000

Penned by Ed Cobb, a member of the clean-cut '50s pop group the Four Preps, Soft Cell twisted the original into a seedy, sleazy masterpiece which, some claim, is impossible to dance to in time.

Soft Cell came to prominence via Stevo's seminal *Some Bizzarre* album, which also featured artists such as Depeche Mode and Blancmange. The Leeds art students Marc Almond and Dave Ball were the first from this record to hit the top spot.

Their debut single, 'Memorabilia', produced by future Mute Records supremo Daniel Miller, had failed to chart. But when the duo reworked the Gloria Jones northern soul classic, 'Tainted Love', the public bought the record in their droves. The song hit the No. 1 spot in a dozen countries and spent a record-breaking 43 weeks in the US *Billboard* charts on its way to a Top Ten slot (a full six months after its UK success).

Soft Cell quickly became associated with the New Romantic movement, despite having little in common with groups such as Duran Duran and Spandau Ballet. Their more quirky and enigmatic sound is now seen as highly influential and was at its best on the 1982 album *Non-Stop Erotic Cabaret*. In 2001, shock

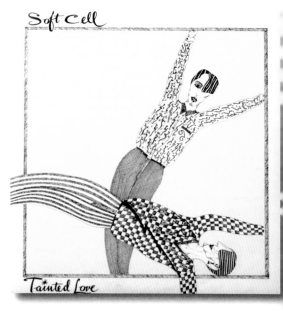

rocker Marilyn Manson returned 'Tainted Love' to the Top Ten with his own goth-rock version from the soundtrack to *Scary Movie 2*.

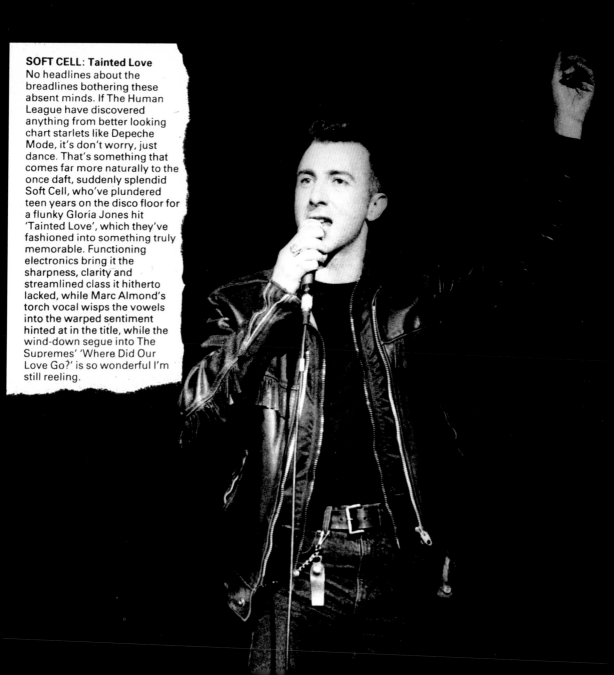

SOFT CELL: Tainted Love
No headlines about the breadlines bothering these absent minds. If The Human League have discovered anything from better looking chart starlets like Depeche Mode, it's don't worry, just dance. That's something that comes far more naturally to the once daft, suddenly splendid Soft Cell, who've plundered teen years on the disco floor for a flunky Gloria Jones hit 'Tainted Love', which they've fashioned into something truly memorable. Functioning electronics bring it the sharpness, clarity and streamlined class it hitherto lacked, while Marc Almond's torch vocal wisps the vowels into the warped sentiment hinted at in the title, while the wind-down segue into The Supremes' 'Where Did Our Love Go?' is so wonderful I'm still reeling.

58 Stranger On The Shore
Mr Acker Bilk and His Paramount Jazz Band

Release Date: 30.11.61
No. Weeks In Chart: 55
Reached No. 1: N/A
Total Sales: 1,130,000

Bilk's less glamourous first names of Bernard Stanley were quickly changed to plain Acker, which in his parochial Somerset dialect means 'friend'.

The famously bowler-hatted clarinetist Bilk made for an unlikely bedfellow in the charts with the first generation of rock 'n' rollers. He was at the forefront of a surprise trad-jazz revival in 1961, which introduced a brash New Orleans style of the genre into the pop world. The catch phrase of the year was 'It's trad, Dad!' and Bilk enjoyed this, his biggest hit, as a result. This, his seventh single, came after previously mixed chart success but remained in the charts for a year. It never reached the hallowed No. 1 spot, but sold well over one million copies.

Acker Bilk had learned to play the clarinet while in the Royal Engineers, and then went on to polish off his talents on the instrument while imprisoned by the army for sleeping on duty.

Jazz mythology has it that Bilk attributed his instantly recognisable style of clarinet playing to two injuries: the loss of two of his front teeth in a schoolyard fight and the loss of the tip of his finger, which was sliced off in a sledding mishap.

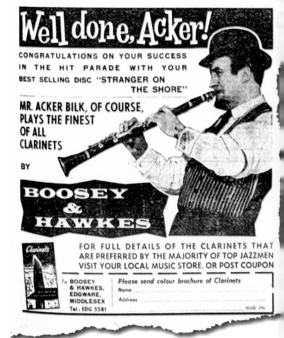

In America, keyboardist Dave Brubeck had introduced jazz into the mainstream and Bilk, along with Kenny Ball, subsequently enjoyed Top Five hits in that country as well. 'Stranger on the Shore' out-stripped its performance in the UK, giving Bilk a US No. 1.

At the height of their appeal, Bilk and his Paramount Jazz band even starred in their own film, *Bank of Thieves*. But then the twist came along and stifled the trad-jazz revival. Bilk enjoyed a return to the charts in 1976 with 'Aria'.

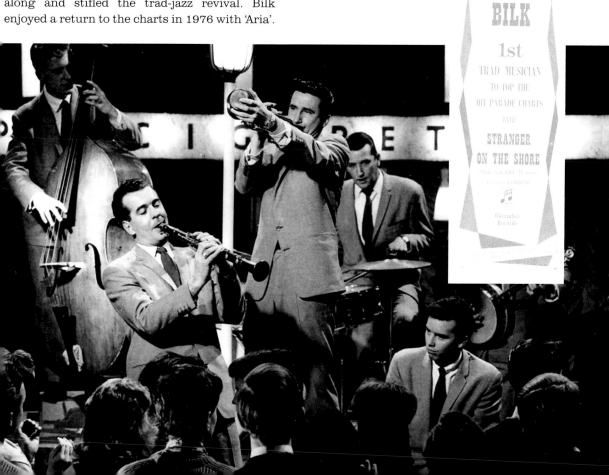

Congratulations

Mr. ACKER BILK

1st

TRAD MUSICIAN TO TOP THE HIT PARADE CHARTS WITH

STRANGER ON THE SHORE

Columbia Records

59 It's Like That
Run-D.M.C. vs Jason Nevins

Release Date: 21.03.98
No. Weeks In Chart: 20
Reached No. 1: 21.03.98
Total Sales: 1,119,905

Nevins cleverly speeded up Run-D.M.C.'s 1983 US-only debut to make it appeal to house-music fans.

This ultra-cool remix was released amid a huge revival in the commercial fortunes of hip-hop. Although novelty remixes of the Beastie Boys' 'Fight For Your Right' had seen similar Top 20 success in this year, Nevins' credentials were impeccable.

A graphic design student who started DJ-ing at college radio in Arizona, Nevins soon moved on to recording tracks for compilation albums and released his first, self-titled EP in 1994. Nevins' debut album, *Green*, was released the following year and he soon found himself remixing for stars such as Janet Jackson and Lil' Kim.

His inspired decision to speed up Run-D.M.C.'s 1983 US-only debut made the Nevins track the ideal offering for house music fans, and this dovetailed perfectly with the prevailing atmosphere in pop music at the time, which saw a return to old-school hip-hop; all this against a tiresome backdrop of clichéd gangsta-rap and excessive commercialism in the genre.

The resulting million-seller (which seeped in at first through import) went straight into the UK charts at No. 1 and kept the Spice Girls'

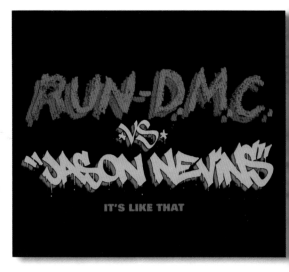

'Stop' off the top slot, giving Run-D.M.C. their first Top 40 hit in over a decade. The single also topped the charts across Europe, adding worldwide sales of another two million copies to this UK total.

Nevins' subsequent work has reflected his affection for hits of the '80s and has included remixes of Run-D.M.C.'s 'It's Tricky' and Toni Basil's 'Mickey'.

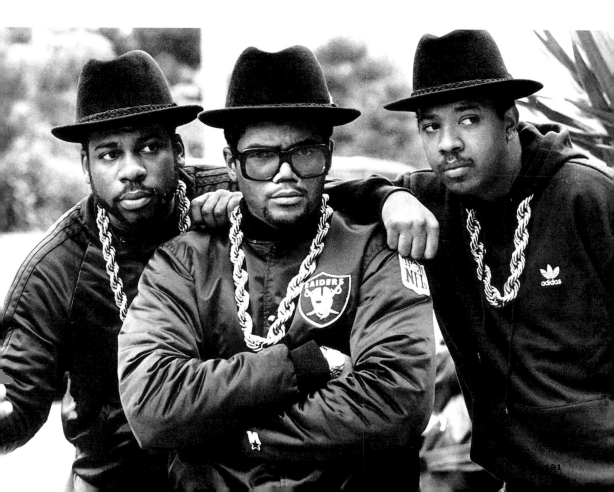

60 Teletubbies Say Eh-Oh
Teletubbies

Release Date: 13.12.97
No. Weeks In Chart: 32
Reached No 1: 13.12.97
Total Sales: 1,107,235

One of the biggest children's programmes in British TV history produced this No. 1 hit.

The Teletubbies were launched in 1997 on the BBC network to appeal to a specific and extremely narrow television-viewing market – the previously largely ignored one- to four-year-old group.

Anne Wood and Andrew Davenport of Ragdoll Limited collated exhaustive market research via a series of focus groups involving nursery-school children.

Every element of the tiny tots' language was analysed – for, even though they may sound strangely alien to grown-up ears, the Teletubbies' bizarre language and odd vocal noises closely mirror very young children's rudimentary speech and linguistic patterns. (When the show was first aired, its makers were accused by some of dumbing down because the characters didn't 'talk' in a conventional sense.)

The brightly coloured creatures – Tinky Winky, Dipsy, Laa-Laa and Po – can each transmit television pictures on their tummies. They live in Teletubbyland, a rather thinly populated world with the odd rabbit and a paranoid hoover, probably unsettled by the fact that the sun appears to contain a baby's face.

However bizarre the Teletubbies might appear to adult eyes, however, the brilliantly conceived show was a huge smash – *Teletubbies* soon became the must-have children's toy, and extensive merchandising proved a big hit. A media storm over the 'sexuality' of the handbag-carrying Tinky Winky and novelty popularity with students – for whom the show's surreal overtones and colourful imagery held a strong appeal – helped to lift the single's profile still further.

This No. 1 hit was only kept from the Christmas top spot by the Spice Girls at their peak (with their single 'Too Much').

The Teletubbies' 1998 US airing was a similar success story, although Christian leader Jerry Falwell re-ignited the controversy over Tinky Winky's sexual orientation.

The programme has since been made into 365 episodes, translated into 35 languages and screened in over 80 countries. Prompted by the success of 'Teletubbies say Eh-Oh', three albums were subsequently released, *Nursery Rhymes and Other Fun Songs!*, *Bedtime and Play Stories* and *Go! Exercise with the Teletubbies* . . . Video sales in 1999 alone were in excess of five million.

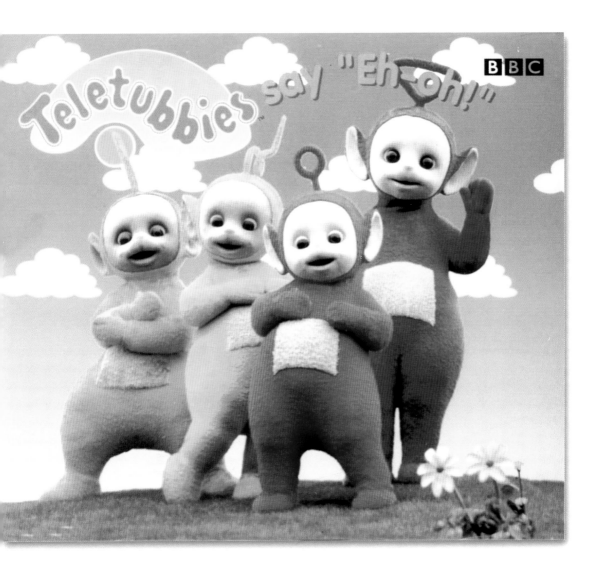

61 Babylon Zoo
Spaceman

Release Date: 27.01.96
No. Weeks In Chart: 14
Reached No. 1: 27.01.96
Total Sales: 1,098,880

The Levi's jeans advertisement that used the song actually aired a snippet of the speeded-up Arthur Baker remix, which served as an introduction for the rather more pedestrian original version.

One of several tracks in this list to be buoyed by their association with a major brand, Babylon Zoo's stuttering attempts to launch their career finally exploded in record-breaking style with this, the biggest-selling single of 1996.

Centred on the enigmatic nucleus of Jas Mann, from Dudley in the West Midlands, Babylon Zoo had emerged from the embers of their indie predecessors The Sandkings, who enjoyed brief success supporting the Stone Roses and Happy Mondays on tour.

'Spaceman' was anything but 'indie' – a glam-rock beast that sold just under 1.1 million copies at the start of 1996, becoming the then fastest-selling debut record in UK chart history. Unfortunately consigned to the record books as a one-hit wonder (his subsequent album *The Boy with the X-Ray Eyes* failed to sell heavily), Mann remains a sharply talented musician who has perhaps been suffocated by the sheer enormity of his breakthrough song.

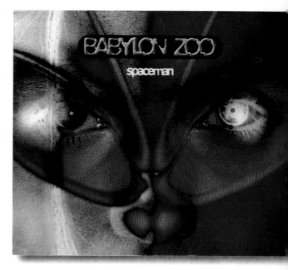

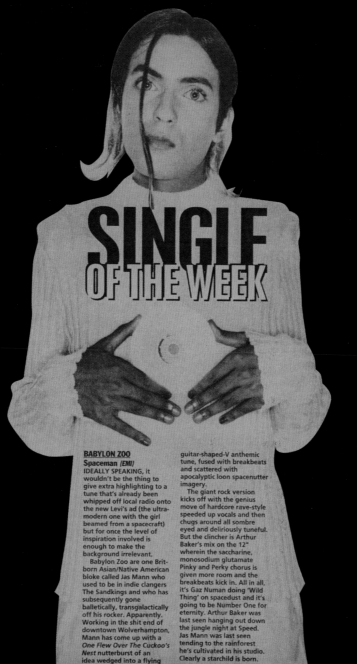

SINGLE
OF THE WEEK

BABYLON ZOO
Spaceman *(EMI)*

IDEALLY SPEAKING, it wouldn't be the thing to give extra highlighting to a tune that's already been whipped off local radio onto the new Levi's ad (the ultra-modern one with the girl beamed from a spacecraft) but for once the level of inspiration involved is enough to make the background irrelevant.

Babylon Zoo are one Brit-born Asian/Native American bloke called Jas Mann who used to be in indie clangers The Sandkings and who has subsequently gone balletically, transgalactically off his rocker. Apparently. Working in the shit end of downtown Wolverhampton, Mann has come up with a *One Flew Over The Cuckoo's Nest* nutterburst of an idea wedged into a flying guitar-shaped-V anthemic tune, fused with breakbeats and scattered with apocalyptic loon spacenutter imagery.

The giant rock version kicks off with the genius move of hardcore rave-style speeded up vocals and then chugs around all sombre eyed and deliriously tuneful. But the clincher is Arthur Baker's mix on the 12" wherein the saccharine, monosodium glutamate Pinky and Perky chorus is given more room and the breakbeats kick in. All in all, it's Gaz Numan doing 'Wild Thing' on spacedust and it's going to be Number One for eternity. Arthur Baker was last seen hanging out down the jungle night at Speed. Jas Mann was last seen tending to the rainforest he's cultivated in his studio. Clearly a starchild is born.

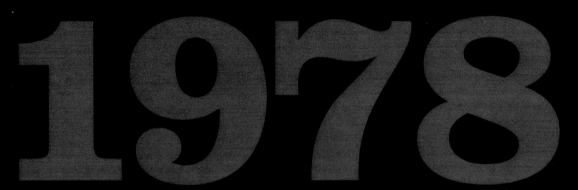

1978

The year 1978 is featured here because it is unique in this book. It is the only year to enjoy multiple entries in the Top Ten list of best-selling singles ever.

In total, the year 1978 boasts six entries in this book, with just under ten million sales between them, contributing significantly to that year's grand total of over 100 million singles sold.

There were some dreadful world events in 1978. Californian Congressman Leo Ryan was killed by the Reverend Jim Jones, who then called for the cyanide suicide of 900 converts to his People's Temple cult (Jones killed himself with a gunshot); the Jonestown Massacre remains one of the worst instances of mass suicide on record. Even more grisly events were exposed when a Vietnamese invasion of Cambodia revealed the true horror of the Khmer Rouge's genocide, with the discovery of mass graves filled with the bodies of hundreds of thousands of opponents and innocent civilians. In March, a devastating oil spill saw 1.3 million barrels of crude oil bleed into the coast of Brittany, France.

On a more positive note, it seemed that Aldous Huxley's 1932 novel, *Brave New World*, in which he predicted babies being made in laboratories, was not just science fiction. On 26 July 1978, it was announced that the world's

1978 NME READER

● For results analysis, see page 26

EST MALE SINGER

David Bowie
John Lydon
Elvis Costello
ob Geldof
on Anderson
e Strummer
Dury
ert Plant
l Weller
e Shelley
ce Springsteen
r Gabriel
Dylan
Jagger
Daltrey

FEMALE
R

arry
Sioux
h
ene
enetration)
trading

eet

dt
on

the Jam
Rope —
s — Thin

ouxsie &

— Elvis

SINGLE

1 White Man In Hammersmith Palais — The Clash
2 Public Image — Public Image Ltd
3 Rat Trap — The Boomtown Rats
4 Down In The Tube Station At Midnight — The Jam
5 Hong Kong Garden — Siouxsie & The Banshees
6 Shot By Both Sides — Magazine
7 Miss You — Rolling Stones
8 Because The Night — Patti Smith Group
9 Jilted John — Jilted John
10 Baker Street — Gerry Rafferty

SONGWRITER

1 Elvis Costello
2 Paul Weller
3 David Bowie
4 Strummer/Jones
5 Pete Shelley
6 Bob Dylan
7 Bob Geldof
8 Bruce Springsteen
9 Ian Dury
10 Anderson / Squire / Howe

BEST DRESSED SLEEVE

1 Some Girls — The Rolling Stones
2 Live & Dangerous — Thin Lizzy
3 Giv...

BEST GROUP

1 The Clash
2 The Jam
3 The Boomtown Rats
4 Genesis
5 Buzzcocks
6 The Stranglers
7 Thin Lizzy
8 The Rolling Stones
9 Yes
10 Siouxsie & The Banshees
11 Led Zeppelin
12 Elvis Costello & The Attractions
13 The Who
14 Ian Dury & The Blockheads
15 Queen
16 Tom Robinson Band
17 Graham Parker & The Rumour
18 Blondie
19 Electric Light Orchestra
20 Status Quo

BEST NEW GROUP

1 Public Image Ltd
2 Stiff Little Fingers
3 Siouxsie & The Banshees
4 Dire Straits
5 The Cars
6 The Undertones
7 The Boomtown Rats
8 John Cooper-Clarke
9 Magazine
10 Van Halen
11 Devo
12 Penetration
13 Th...

KEYBOARDS

1 Dave Greenfield
2 Rick Wakeman
3 Johnny Fingers
4 Tony Banks
5 Brian Eno
6 Steve Naive
7 Keith Emerson
8 Barry Andrews
9 Dave Formula
10 Jon Lord

DRUMS

1 Keith Moon
2 John Maher
3 Topper Headon
4 Phil Collins
5 Rick Buckler
6 Charlie Watts
7 Kenny Morris
8 Cozy Powell
9 Jet Black
10 Brian Downey

DJ

1 John Peel
2 Anne Nightingale
3 Kenny Everett
4 Nicky Horne
5 Noel Edmonds
6 Alan Freeman
7 Kid Jensen
8 Dave Lee Travis
9 Roger Scott
10 Simon Bates

RADIO SHOW

1 John P...

197

first test tube baby, Louise Brown, had been born in Oldham District Hospital (the fertilisation was actually performed in a shallow glass dish, not a test tube).

In the world of entertainment, the year saw the debut of the musical *Evita*, the film *The Deer Hunter* and the first *Superman* blockbuster. On television, *Sale of the Century*, *George and Mildred*, *Taxi* and *Dallas* reigned supreme. Ultrasound was first used, jogging became something of a national craze, Space Invader arcade games captivated young kids everywhere, martial law was introduced in Iran under the Shah and the Turin Shroud was presented as a bona fide biblical artefact. The year also saw three different popes and . . . disco (no correlation).

Disco was the most obvious chart hit of 1978. The massive box-office success of *Saturday Night Fever* made John Travolta a mega-star and also revived the careers of the Bee Gees, who then reached a new peak. The Lancashire-bred band had not made much impact on the UK charts since 1972, although they had enjoyed some US success, but the soundtrack to one of the year's two biggest films rocketed them back to global fame.

Although *Saturday Night Fever* was the stylistic hit of the celluloid year and provided the best-selling album of 1978, it was the second Travolta vehicle, *Grease*, which enjoyed more single success. Although six of the songs from the Bee Gees' *Saturday Night Fever* soundtrack made No. 1, none could compete with the huge sales of 'You're The One That I Want' and 'Summer Nights' (see No.'s 6 and 21).

However, the retro look of *Grease* never really trickled into the high-street clothes stores. Instead, it was the white flared suits and glitzy clothes of the disco world that made their indelible mark, not least on the covers of numerous disco compilation albums – perhaps most famously on those released by K-Tel.

The year had started off with Wings' 'Mull O' Kintyre' still on top of the charts, where it enjoyed a total of nine weeks at No. 1 (see No. 4). Entries in this list that were actually released in 1978 include the tongue-in-cheek camp extravaganza of The Village People (see No. 33), which was in stark contrast to the underground cool of fellow chart-topper, Ian Dury (see No. 87).

Elsewhere, The Police and The Jam were starting to make waves in a year that also saw the Sex Pistols and The Damned disband. Johnny Rotten reverted to John Lydon and unveiled Public Image Limited, while Sid Vicious was arrested on the charge of murdering his girlfriend Nancy Spungen in a New York Hotel – Sid himself was dead within four months.

Although punk still infected the mainstream – even seeing a film of its life in *Jubilee* – the underground potency and cultural freshness had evaporated (Paul McCartney was rumoured to have decided against releasing a 'punk' single called 'Boil Crisis'). Another of the big chart names of the year was Darts, with smash singles such as 'Come Back My Love' and 'Boy From New York City'. The Commodores' 'Three Times A Lady' was also a huge hit; 10 CC's 'Dreadlock Holiday' enjoyed one week at No. 1

The huge singles sales of 1978 can perhaps be attributed to several factors. Punk and New Wave bands had opened up a new market releasing coloured vinyl and collectible formats, with the twelve-inch single becoming a firm favourite, especially in the dance market.

The pinnacle of these historically high sales (1978 jumped up 30 per cent on 1977) was Boney M's 'Rivers of Babylon', with demand being so colossal that UK pressing plants could not cope (see No. 5). Kate Bush hit the top with her debut 'Wuthering Heights'; Abba appeared in their own film; and there was also room for the odd novelty hit, such as Brian and Michael's homage to the artist Lowry, 'Matchstalk Men and Matchstalk Cats and Dogs'.

Two other years have enjoyed greater sales within the context of this list – 1984's six entries grossed over 10.5 million sales, while the biggest tally is 1997's near-thirteen million copies from seven entries. Yet it is 1978, with its gold lamé, white flares, crumbling punk scene, all-conquering soundtracks and T Birds, which provides a plethora of classic snapshots imprinted on the cultural memory.

Well, apart from Leo Sayer.

THE SATURDAY NIGHT FEVER INDUSTRY

THE STARTLING RISE to popularity of *Saturday Night Fever* has been widely portrayed as a traditional success story — the rise of a brand new superstar in the form of John Travolta, whose mugshot currently adorns the front covers of publications as adverse as U.S. gossip rag *The Star* and the political heavyweight *Time*.

Far more interesting in many ways, however, is the story of how *Fever* was developed into a media goldmine which is now, according to *Variety*, "building into a music industry all by itself".

As *Thrills* predicted in January, music movies have come of age with a vengeance in 1978. In recent weeks in America, *Fever* has topped the film charts, the album charts *and* the tape charts, with five tracks from the album taking up no less than *half* the U.S. Top Ten singles in one recent week.

The financial facts are staggering. Leaving aside the astronomical amounts of money the movie itself is grossing, the album has already sold 6 million copies, and is now selling at the rate of a million copies a week, with a projected final sale in sight of 12 million copies — which would make the double record set the biggest grossing album of all time. (*The Sound of Music* is still holding the record for biggest selling soundtrack album at 16 million copies to date, but that is only a single album).

All the album tracks (The Bee Gees and other RSO artists aside) were licensed from other companies on a deal which means that if *Fever* does reach the 12 million mark, the licensees will walk away with a cool $360,000 per track.

For those artists

is now poised to become one of the most powerful figures in the music business.

Saturday Night Fever was handled with consummate marketing skill. This was no word-of-mouth movie. Travolta was already a small screen star via his Fonzie-like role in the American TV sitcom *Welcome Back Kotter*. This, combined with the movie's eminently commercial disco music, backed by some extremely hard-sell advertising techniques, enabled the package to scale new financial heights of *Jaws*-like proportions.

Having successfully launched the film via a massive in-cinema campaign, the Stigwood organisation went on to spend a phenomenal amount on TV advertising for the album — a quarter of a million dollars in Europe alone.

This reflects current industry trends — movies sell albums and singles, which in turn sell movies. Soundtrack albums dominated the recent Grammy awards (America's music biz equivalent of Oscars), and are currently making huge dents in the 'straight' album market. Biggies to date are the two *Star Wars* albums (soundtrack and spoken word) and *Close Encounters*, all of which are currently approaching platinum status.

Nobody understands this present shift in the industry better than Robert Stigwood, and he is now about to capitalise on it in a way that is going to make even the *Fever* earnings look like chicken feed.

For a start, he has two more major music movies all ready for release later this year. First will be *Grease*, an *American Graffiti* style '50s pastiche based on a long-running Broadway smash, which once again stars John Travolta, this time teamed with Olivia John.

62 I Remember You
Frank Ifield

Release Date: 5.07.62
No. Weeks In Chart: 28
Reached No. 1: 26.07.62
Total Sales: 1,096,000

Ifield was the first artist to achieve three consecutive No. 1 hits in Britain and also the first to be awarded three gold discs in the same year.

Coventry-born Ifield is most readily associated with Australia, where he was brought up and enjoyed early career success. His first Australian record was made when he was aged thirteen, but after 44 releases Down Under as a radio star, Ifield gambled on a career in the UK and moved here in 1959.

After two modest releases, his revival of Jimmy Dorsey's 1942 song 'I Remember You' hit No. 1, where it stayed for two months, also bringing him US debut chart success (in the Top Five). 1962 was the year for his country-style, yodel-influenced vocals and clean-cut image, with 'Lovesick Blues' and 'The Wayward Wind' also hitting the top spot (complemented by his own TV programme, *The Frank Ifield Show*). Only Cliff Richard and Elvis were more successful that year.

An almost relentless touring schedule over 25 years kicked off with early support slots being taken by The Beatles. His other most famous song, the Australian standard 'Waltzing Matilda', was never actually a single although Ifield's version is regarded as definitive.

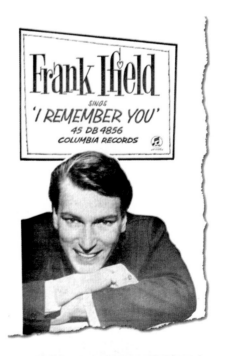

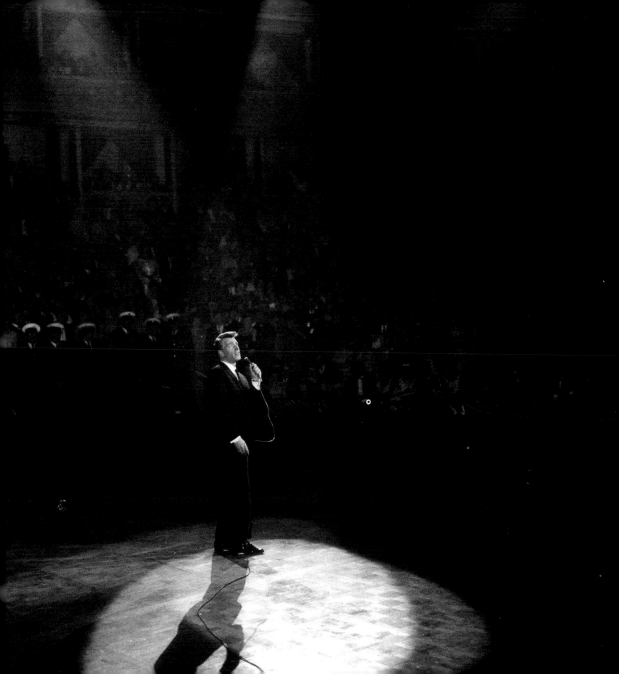

63 I Believe/Up On The Roof
Robson and Jerome

Release Date: 11.11.95
No. Weeks In Chart: 14
Reached No. 1: 11.11.95
Total Sales: 1,093,972

As with all three of the duo's singles, this track went straight in at the No. 1 slot.

Capitalising on the nostalgic and record-breaking success of their debut single (see No. 9), Robson Green and Jerome Flynn enjoyed another million-seller with this cover version of 'I Believe'.

Seemingly immune to the meteoric rise of Britpop and the Blur vs Oasis battles going on in the charts, sales of the pair's second single were as startling as the first. As with all three of their singles (the third was 'What Becomes of the Broken Hearted'), this track went straight in at No. 1 and stayed there for a full month.

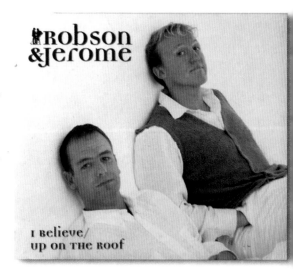

Their debut album sold even more – a remarkable 1.85 million copies, securing the No. 1 slot for nearly two months – and a long-form video did proportionately good business, too. At the peak of their brief omnipresence in the UK charts, they were even presented to the Queen at the Royal Variety Show.

Robson has since founded Coastal Productions, a drama outfit aimed at providing support and encouragement to youngsters who want to get into drama in the north-east of England. Both Robson and Jerome have gone on to establish themselves as two of British television's most popular actors.

ROBSON & JEROME
I Believe *(RCA)*

AS NIKE might say, just duet.

Robson and Jerome, who will forever be known as "those two twats off *Soldier Soldier* who kept 'Common People' stuck at Number Two, the bastards", make a somewhat premature bid for the Christmas Number One slot with the full range of sweeping strings and strangely homoerotic sentiments, cooing *"I believe for every drop of rain that falls, our flower grows"* in each other's ears. Steady on now lads please, that sort of thing isn't allowed in the Army just yet.

64 Saturday Night
Whigfield

Release Date: 17.09.94
No. Weeks In Chart: 18
Reached No. 1: 17.09.94
Total Sales: 1,092,250

Deliberately targeting the UK's millions of 'Brits Abroad' clubbers, the track was a huge summer party anthem in Spanish nightclubs and in the UK home territory, too.

Former model-turned-pop star Whigfield started life as Sannie Charlotte Carlson in her Danish hometown of Skaelskar, before moving to the Ivory Coast and then Italy with her jazz-loving parents. After a stint as a waitress and a school cleaner, she enrolled at fashion college before turning to modelling. However, she became painfully thin and uneasy with the oppressive world of the catwalk, so began to study music and sing in a band with her brother.

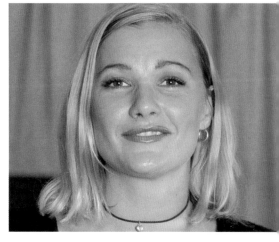

Taking the moniker 'Whigfield' from her favourite teacher, Carlson met up with producer Larry Pignagnoli, who had already helped launch Spagna. 'Saturday Night' sold nearly 1.1 million of its total of three million copies in the UK alone (the first territory where it was No. 1), in the process knocking the record-breaking 'Love Is All Around' by Wet Wet Wet off the top position (see No. 11).

A four-week stay was buoyed by second-week sales which were the highest for any artist since Band Aid (see No. 2). Whigfield hardly maintained the Scandinavian musical legacy left by Abba (although the latter are not represented in this list), but nonetheless did replicate, to a degree, the commercial success of artists such as Roxette and Ace of Base.

Cover versions by The Smurfs and the plastic doll Sindy have done little to increase the kudos of the original. Subsequent Whigfield singles gradually slipped further down the charts, until a 1998 release missed the Top 40 altogether.

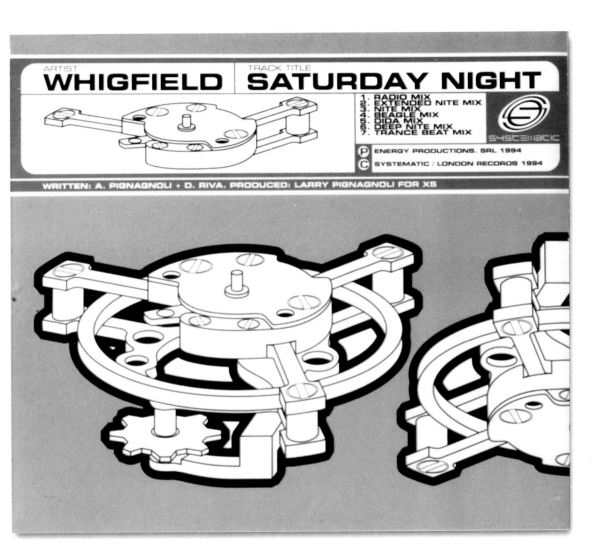

ARTIST
WHIGFIELD

TRACK TITLE
SATURDAY NIGHT

1. RADIO MIX
2. EXTENDED NITE MIX
3. NITE MIX
4. BEAGLE MIX
5. DIDA MIX
6. DEEP NITE MIX
7. TRANCE BEAT MIX

systematic

℗ ENERGY PRODUCTIONS. SRL 1994
© SYSTEMATIC / LONDON RECORDS 1994

WRITTEN: A. PIGNAGNOLI + D. RIVA. PRODUCED: LARRY PIGNAGNOLI FOR XS

65 Pure & Simple
Hear'Say

Release Date:	24.03.01
No. Weeks In Chart:	25
Reached No. 1:	24.03.01
Total Sales:	1,078,434

The sight of 10,000 hopefuls queuing for their fifteen seconds of fame and caustic scorn from the judges proved unmissable television and fantastic record-company PR.

Hear'Say is the tabloid lovechild of TV ratings winner *Pop Stars* and the public's seemingly insatiable appetite for celebrity. Their debut single, 'Pure & Simple', was the then fastest-selling single in British chart history (only superseded by *Pop Idol* winner, Will Young – see No. 12).

While the scorn from the judges – led by *übermeister* 'Nasty Nigel' Lythgoe – made compelling viewing, the commercial impact of continual prime-time TV exposure only began to manifest itself when record stores started to report staggering advance orders. Secrecy over the identities of the five winners and the lead single itself whipped the nation into a frenzy and made 'Pure & Simple' a guaranteed chart topper (first-day sales alone exceeded 160,000).

In doing so, it kept Westlife's charity Red Nose single 'Uptown Girl' off the No. 1 slot. The accompanying album, *Pop Stars*, was a simultaneous album chart-topper, the first time a debut single and debut album reached the top at the same time. However, Hear'Say proved unable to sustain this level of success – their

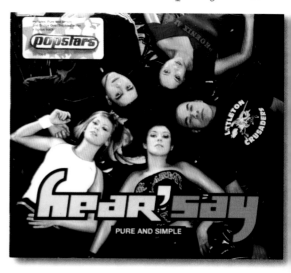

second single sold only 16,000 on its first day. A disastrous second album, cancelled tours and the departure of Kym Marsh for a solo career exacerbated the band's problems. Even runners-up and 'Flop Stars', Liberty X, enjoyed more credibility and eventual chart-topping success. In October 2002, the remaining Hear'Say members announced their decision to split.

Hear'Say

Pure And Simple *(Polydor)*

How bad did you expect your postmodern pop experiment to be? Wrong, it's much, much worse. This isn't even a song, it's just one long fade-out from All Saints 'Never Ever' on a loop, pure and fucking simple. Hey Darius, you were lucky pal. Only a drug bust or suicide can possibly make them interesting again. That sound, Hear'Say, is Atomic Kitten and Sugababes *laughing* at you

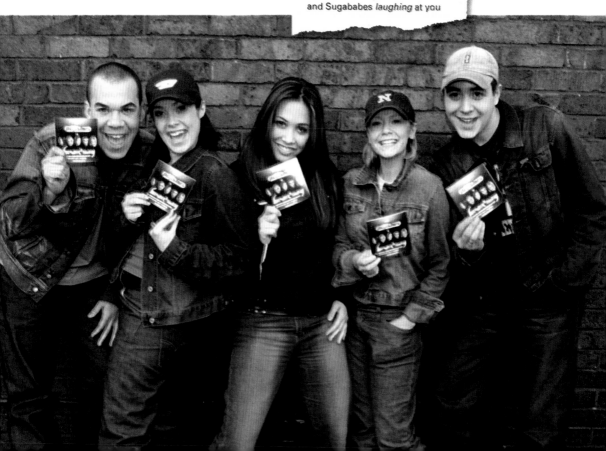

66 No Matter What
Boyzone

Release Date: 15.08.98

No. Weeks In Chart: 15

Reached No. 1: 15.08.98

Total Sales: 1,074,192

Despite early critical pillorying, Boyzone enjoyed a meteoric rise to fame and a lengthy run of Top Five hits.

Plucked from Dublin's Northside by notable pop manager Louis Walsh, Boyzone brashly seized Take That's crown on the latter's 1996 demise. One of the audition songs sung by Ronan Keating, Keith Duffy, Shane Lynch and Stephen Gateley was George Michael's 'Careless Whisper' (see No. 34).

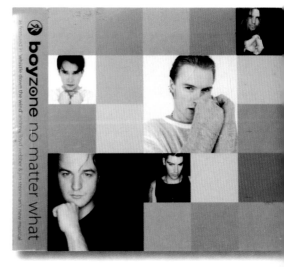

The group's inauspicious start took the shape of a rather muted TV performance the day after they had first formed. The departure of two original members brought in Mikey Graham. Keating then abandoned a New York athletics college course and Olympic aspirations to cement the line-up.

In the pre-Spice Girls era, Boyzone enjoyed a meteoric rise to fame – in the early days, Keating was still working in a shoe shop. An Irish-only hit with the somewhat dubious 'Working My Way Back To You' preceded their first UK single, 'Love Me For A Reason', which hit No. 2. From there on, the group enjoyed a further fifteen straight Top Five UK hits.

The band first performed this, their best-selling track, at Andrew Lloyd Webber's 50th birthday party. It was their fourth No. 1 and came six months after Keating had lost his mother, grandmother and teenage cousin all within the space of twelve weeks.

Plagued by rumours of a split and inter-band animosity for much of their career, the band has been inactive since 2000, although Gately's coming out as a homosexual and modest solo efforts from all but Keating have kept their profile high. Keating also went on to manage chart sensation Westlife.

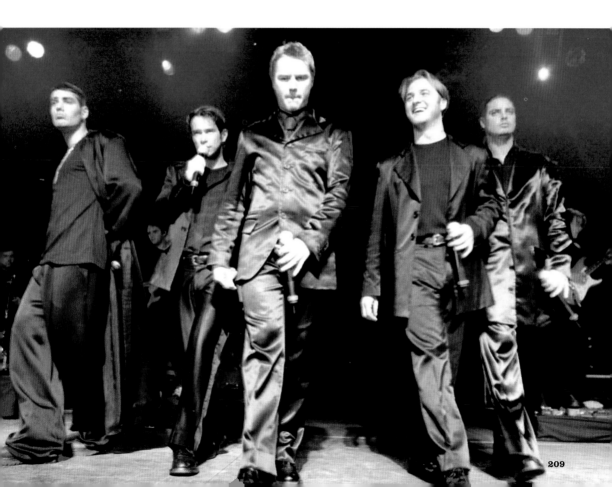

Censorship and Music

" I know this man is dangerous and I don't want to see British youngsters hacking out his name on their arms . . . or see sex treated as an appalling commercial freak show.'

An English reporter voices his concerns after the 1956 release of Elvis Presley's 'Hound Dog'

Censorship has never stifled music. It feeds music. One band perhaps more than any other perfectly represents the ongoing battle between the moral majority and their musical nemesis: the Sex Pistols. In the short term, the Sex Pistols were inconvenienced by censorship; in the long term it was invaluable in helping to cement their legend.

Railing against massive rock gods such as Led Zeppelin, Genesis, Pink Floyd et al and the monster that was prog-rock, the Pistols' short, sharp, shock treatment appalled even rock's most liberal diehards. The catalyst was a shop called 'Sex' on the King's Road in Chelsea, west London, itself a one-time bastion of all things unconventional. The outrageous sartorial genius of the duo Vivienne Westwood and Malcolm McLaren swirled around the Pistols, making their anti-social fashion statements indiscernible from their confrontational music.

The band's debut single, 'Anarchy In The UK', is a seismic snapshot of what was about to happen. Swearing on a live TV show led to some of the most vitriolic scorn and establishment horror ever poured on a musical outfit, all soaked up with vigour and spat back at the

PARENTAL
ADVISORY
EXPLICIT CONTENT

horrified and staid British public. From there, the Pistols rapidly became the band of the moment with their high-profile stunts (signing a record deal outside Buckingham Palace), their abrasive records (recommended listening? All of it) and their incendiary live shows (prone to violence, guaranteed to be memorable). Soon, the authorities were – allegedly – conspiring to keep their releases from the No.1 spot, holding the top slot free instead for old favourites like Rod Stewart.

To a new-millennial teenager drip-fed on Blink 182 and Limp Bizkit, the Sex Pistols' music may even sound tame, certainly dated. The point here is context. When the Pistols released 'God Save The Queen' in the summer of 1977, as the UK basked in a heat wave and enjoyed street parties to celebrate the Queen's 25th Silver Jubilee, there could have been no greater anti-establishment statement.

When the Pistols hired a boat, the *Queen Elizabeth*, to launch the single, they soon found themselves at the centre of a near-riot when they tried to disembark on the banks of the River Thames. The Pistols knew how to cause an almighty stink.

They also knew how to maximise any censorship that came their way – and there was plenty of it. Venues refused to stage agreed gigs, magazines pulled articles, TV stations refused entry to their premises and radio stations blanked them. Furthermore, if the censors hated the Sex Pistols, they loathed Sid Vicious. Censorship thrives by demonising individuals – more recently, Eminem, Marilyn Manson and Trent Reznor – but their outraged words fell on deaf ears when they denounced Sid. Vicious, called to arms to replace the founder bassist, Glen Matlock, soon became the living, breathing epitome of everything that punk rock stood for.

He was hated, loathed, loved and adored. His own personal story ended in a swathe of hard drugs, a murder charge and eventual – fatal – drugs overdose at the age of 22. It was a modern tragedy played out on the pages of music newspapers who themselves enjoyed a new lease of life chronicling the phenomenon.

Sid was a triumph of attitude over ability. He taught himself the rudiments of bass in one night and joined the band he loved to watch play. It was said that he was into David Bowie and Marc Bolan, wearing sandals and painting his toenails – when he couldn't get his hair to stand up like Bowie's, he put his head in an oven to bake it into place.

His short-lived career was fuelled by colossal drug binges, violence and an insane touring lifestyle. Sid blurred the edges between seemingly immortal punk myth and the reality of dole queues, benefits and isolation. When he was in hospital in early 1978, Sid admitted to one photographer, 'My basic nature is going to kill me within six months.' He was wrong, but only by half a year.

The Pistols, unbelievably, only made one album. They lasted only around two years from their absurd, raucous beginnings at St Martin's College (when the plug was pulled on them after a handful of songs) to their ramshackle finale at Winterland in San Francisco. By then so many authorities were threatening venues

...hat touring had become a near-impossibility. When the Sex Pistols finally imploded, the censors would have struggled to muffle their smug self-congratulation, but the snarling beast that had turned British popular culture on its head would have the last laugh.

Of course, censorship in music did not start with the Sex Pistols. Way back in 1951, Dean Martin's song, 'Wham Bam, Thank You Ma'am', was the subject of widespread complaint and restricted availability due to what were perceived as 'suggestive' lyrics.

At one point in the '50s, jukeboxes were banned within hearing distance of churches in some of America's southern states. The unlikely looking Bill Haley (see No. 31) was at the centre of much criticism and attempted censorship when his 'anti-establishment' teen film *Rock Around The Clock* apparently 'caused' riots in London's Trocadero cinema at the Elephant and Castle. Some observers admitted later that they had mistaken dancing youngsters for rioters.

'The King' was also a target for censors. A mid-1956 tour was undertaken with the warning that if Elvis-the-Pelvis moved his lower body at all, he would be arrested on obscenity charges. A year later this censure was repeated in an internal memo to the cameramen on *The Ed Sullivan Show*, ordering them not to film below the waist.

Countless songs have been altered, often without an artist's consent, to make them palatable for radio play – John Lennon's 'Working Class Hero' is just one example (see No. 23). Outright bans have been less commonplace, however – perhaps because even the myopic moral majority have spotted the direct correlation between total bans and massive record sales (witness Frankie Goes To Hollywood, see No.'s 7 and 22; also, the furore surrounding The Prodigy's provocatively titled 'Smack My Bitch Up').

It is understandably hard for kids brought up on the violent and sexually explicit music of genres such as gangsta rap to appreciate why The Beatles had the censors in apoplexy. But they did – when John Lennon let slip in an interview that he thought the Fab Four were 'bigger than Jesus', the comment went largely unnoticed in the UK. When it resurfaced some time later in the US, it provoked mass burnings of Beatles' records.

The parental advisory sticker – initially a reaction to a controversial Prince album – has now largely been acknowledged as little more than a useful marketing tool for teasing sales out of curious teens. Elsewhere, failed court actions against numerous metal bands – Ozzy Osbourne and Judas Priest to name but two – have nevertheless tested music's ability to withstand such vocal and well-financed opposition.

Yet, as always, the censors remain undaunted. Even disco music was branded as promoting drug use and criticised for encouraging sexually permissive attitudes. Strangely, the censors let one morally dubious piece of music slip through their otherwise vigilistic net – what damage has been caused to society by Tight Fit's rendering of 'The Lion Sleeps Tonight' is anyone's guess.

67 2 Become 1
Spice Girls

Release Date: 28.12.96
No. Weeks In Chart: 23
Reached No. 1: 28.12.96
Total Sales: 1,072,073

The subtle orchestration and softer tones drew in many older listeners, in the process securing record advance orders of over 750,000 copies.

Buoyed by the lightning-fast sales of their first two releases, the self-acclaimed 'spice squad' enjoyed another enormo-single courtesy of this, their first ballad.

Co-written by the band and the songwriters Stannard/Rowe, the track provided the girls with the first of three consecutive Christmas No. 1s, a success that has been equalled only by The Beatles.

Following the more sexually charged Russ Meyer-like promotional clip for their second outing, 'Say You'll Be There', Baby, Posh, Ginger, Sporty and Scary toned down for a festive jaunt around New York.

Spice Fever had gripped the nation – further supporters were won over by the decision to delay this single release by one week so that the charity and anti-gun campaign record 'Knockin' On Heaven's Door' could enjoy its moment at the top of the charts.

So rapid had been the girls' rise to fame that even before the debut album was released, there were already Spice Girls tribute bands playing the clubs of Britain.

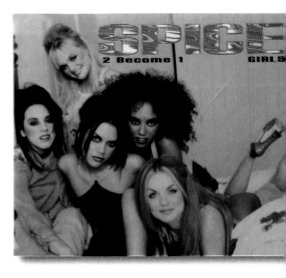

The twilight years of the Spice Girls' career - characterised by acrimonious splits, the merely modest solo success of each group member and the phenomenon of 'Posh and Becks' – should in no way cloud the historical impact of a group who were, in many ways, the quintessential band of the '90s.

SPICE GIRLS
2 Become 1 *(Virgin)*

WHAM! THEY kick your down door with 'Wannabe'. KRAK! They fracture your drooping jaw with 'Say You'll Be There'. SOOTH! You wake up to find them mopping your fevered

SINGLE OF

brow with '2 Become 1'. What? A Spice Girls ballad? Have they lost their balls? Have they sold out? Stop asking such stupid questions. The Spice Girls haven't only conquered pop in 1996, they have redefined it. They ARE pop. To criticise the Spice Girls is thus to attack pop, and to attack pop is to join the still-breathing dead. Look at the opposition – a bunch of Hitler Youth lookalike white guy combos put together by racist scumbag marketing departments to cash in on 'swingbeat' (itself an utterly insipid and worthless genre).

Charlotte Raven, writing in *The Guardian*, snootily mocked Ver Spice for using "feminist signifiers" while lacking any real intellectual muscle to back them up. Duh! They just AM!

THE WEEK

Everybody with half a brain has been arguing for decades that the real power, the real driving force and the real punkyness in the rock/pop thing has always, and will always, be found in the massed ranks of screaming teenage gurlydom. And now, at last, that power has been tapped, refined and encapsulated in the Spice Girls. It may not be the revolution, but 'Girl Power' is easily the most radical slogan spat out by a pop band thus far. Radical, because I've got an eight-year-old mate called Freya who, when she goes to an all-girl party, "saves up her farts" and takes her Spice Girls tapes along with her. Radical because it is believed, acted upon and *lived* by its recipients. The Spice Girls are the best thing to happen in pop for decades and, yes, Sporty Spice is my favourite. Roll over Andrea Dworkin and tell Liam Gallagher the news. Wake up, Britpop, YOU'RE DEAD!

68

The Young Ones
Cliff Richard and The Shadows

Release Date: 11.01.62

No. Weeks In Chart: 21

Reached No. 1: 11.01.62

Total Sales: 1,052,000

An early performance on the TV show, *Oh Boy!*, was reviewed by one pundit as 'violent hip-swinging – a lengthy career [for Cliff] will only be accomplished by dispensing with short-sighted, vulgar antics.'

This is the first of two entries in this book for Sir Cliff, both of them in the '60s with The Shadows (see also No. 90) – perhaps surprising for an artist who has enjoyed hit singles in six separate decades, making him the most successful solo singer in history. This was Indian-born Cliff's fifth No. 1 and his only release to make over one million UK sales. This single had 500,000 advance orders, helped by the movie of the same name, which gave Cliff his first starring role and became the second-biggest box office success of 1962.

Penned by Tepper and Bennett, this single entered at the top and stayed there for six weeks, a feat matched by the film's chart-topping soundtrack album. Despite his relatively lowly position in the list, Cliff is almost without statistical parallel in chart history, with no fewer than 118 Top 40 singles. His most recent No. 1, 'Millennium Prayer', came over 40 years after his first, 'Living Doll'. Cliff infamously re-recorded 'Living Doll', rather than this hit, for the anarchic *The Young Ones* comedy show of 1986.

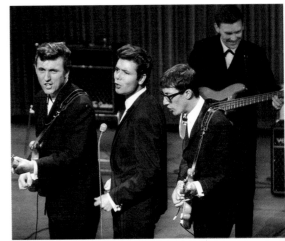

CLIFF joins ELVIS and LONNIE with a No. 1 first-time chart entry!

AND then there were three! Prior to this week, only Elvis Presley and Lonnie Donegan had achieved the fantastic distinction of coming straight into the best-selling lists at the coveted No. 1 position. Now they have been joined by Cliff Richard, who explodes out of the blue to take top spot with " The Young Ones "—a number which was originally planned as the " B " side of the record!

When I talked last week to Norrie Paramor, Cliff's recording manager, he forecast that the disc would make its initial appearance in the No. 1 spot. But Norrie was basing his prophecy on much more than mere optimism. He knew full well that, even before the record was officially released, its orders were fast approaching the half-million mark.

And when I phoned Norrie earlier this week to congratulate him on the amazing success of the record, he told me that the latest sales figures as of Monday evening was 634,900!

So Cliff is certainly well on the way towards winning another Gold Disc!

It could well be that he will secure the rare honour of passing the million mark on the strength of British sales alone. Of course, he is also bound to increase this through handsome sales on the Continent and in the Commonwealth—and, we hope, in the States.

As yet no plans have been made for the release of this disc in America. The record companies are holding fire to assess the position with regard to the film — and I understand that negotiations are currently in hand with an important company in the States for the release of the picture there.

But and when this transpires, it seems highly probable, it's pretty certain that Cliff's recording—and perhaps also the soundtrack LP—will be issued there to coincide with the movie.

Cliff's new record prompts one to reflect upon what might have happened, if his young lad been released as the "B" side. Indeed, in the first place it was not even scheduled for release as a single!

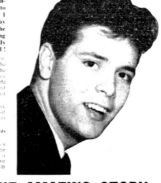

THE AMAZING STORY BEHIND 'YOUNG ONES'

Cliff himself was somewhat dubious about its chances, but he eventually—though rather reluctantly—agreed to its issue, provided that it went out as the "B" side. But after the premiere of the film, at which he was completely bowled over by the overwhelming reception, he changed his mind and gave his blessing to it being switched to the "A" side.

The song, originally planned for January release has now been kept on the shelf to see the light of day at some future date.

One of the most fascinating features of "The Young Ones" single is the unusual effect created by the strings. Norrie Paramor let me into the secret of how this was done—apparently Cliff waxed the song with his usual backing by the Shadows

and the strings were dubbed on to the record afterwards.

"I cribbed this idea from the film," admitted Norrie. "So I must give full credit to Stanley Black, who orchestrated the film score."

But you know, while we are only too ready to congratulate artist and recording manager when their score a triumph of this nature, there's one person who is frequently overlooked —the music publisher. And in this case, I feel that we should pay him special tribute—for without Cyril Simons, of Leeds Music, there wouldn't be a song called "The Young Ones" in existence today.

The story

Here briefly is the story. The basic music score for Cliff's new film was practically complete, though the picture still lacked a title. Cyril, whose company was handling the music, then again suggested that he should commission the celebrated American song team of Topper and Bennett to write a couple of numbers for the movie—including a title song.

His idea was readily accepted and, without further ado he flew off to New York to see the duo in question. You will doubtless recall that Topper and Bennett have previously written a few numbers for Cliff, including his smash hit "Travellin' Light," besides penning songs for such stars as Elvis Presley and Perry Como.

The writers were waiting for Cyril on his arrival in New York. They perused the script together and Cyril left them mulling over it, while he boarded a plane to California for

discussions with Norrie Paramor who was already kicking their at the ready.

Cyril returned to Los Angeles a few hours later, winged straight back to New York, where he found that Topper and Bennett had not only conceived the idea of "The Young Ones," but had a ready-written title song.

In point of fact, they wrote it in a matter of a couple of hours. Surely this was due to the efficient of The Young Ones is the pocket Stephens for you in was eagerly accepted by the film company who had merely found a suitable title for their ambitious new production.

I mentioned just how Cyril had commissioned Topper and Bennett to write two songs for the film. Strangely enough, the other one a just couldn't "Sundust Dreams" was used.

Nevertheless, there was a second Topper and Bennett composition in the movie—the haunting "When The Girl In Your Arms." But this wasn't written specifically for the film.

Indeed, some six months before Cyril's flying visit to the States, they had submitted this song to him through the normal channels in the belief that Cliff might like to record it. Cliff in fact was most impressed and a decision was taken to wax it for release at some future date.

Then, at one of the policy meetings held before the film went into production, it was decided (primarily as a result of Cliff's suggestion) to incorporate it in the picture.

This is just another reason why not only the one song but the entire score of the film is meeting with such

favourable response. And for this we've the duo to thank. Peter Myers and Ronnie Cass, who were responsible for all the scintillating production music in the movie—as well as Norrie Paramor, who wrote the two instrumental items.

Little wonder, therefore, that the soundtrack album is also selling like hot cakes. Latest figure I had from the sales office—which, for an LP is fairly—really some going!

He's on air

How does Cliff feel about the success of his new record? When I talked to him this week he was working on air.

He was just facing a lengthy session at the dentist, but even this didn't shake his enthusiasm.

When we saw the effect of the film we realised that this disc was going to be a big one," he told me. "But this is ridiculous! I just can't believe it. I'm sure the bubble must burst before long."

Cliff mentioned how much he was looking forward to his lengthy six-week tour of one-nighters which begins on January 21. Next week, he's off to Hull, where the Shadows are currently appearing in pantomime, to rehearse some new stage material with them.

"Last week, in my survey of 1961, I pointed out what a marvellous year it had been for British recording artists. Now, with Cliff as their champion and in unbeatable mood it looks as though they are stepping into 1962 on the right foot

69 Earth Song
Michael Jackson

Release Date: 9.12.95
No. Weeks In Chart: 17
Reached No. 1: 9.12.95
Total Sales: 1,038,821

During Jackson's performance of 'Earth Song' at the 1996 Brit Awards, Pulp's Jarvis Cocker infamously ran on stage and wiggled his posterior in protest at what he called Jackson's 'Christ-like' self-opinion.

This is, surprisingly, the only entry for Michael Jackson, an artist who has enjoyed an incredible 48 Top 40 solo UK hits. Ironically, 'Earth Song' is actually one of Jackson's weaker chart successes.

This No. 1 anthemic tirade against humanity's greed and ecological suicide climaxed in a pseudo-Baptist finale by the Andrae Crouch Singers. Backed with a suitably overblown video, the song was the third single taken from the *HIStory* album, Jackson's first since the nadir of child sex-abuse allegations in 1993 (which saw Pepsi withdraw a lucrative sponsorship deal).

The album launch was preceded by a 50-foot statue of the 'King of Pop' being floated under Tower Bridge and up the River Thames. But given the subsequent turn of events, and the gradual slowing down of Jackson's hitherto unstoppable pop momentum, the giant statue was seen by some in hindsight as an act of hubris. It was this same perceived arrogance

that prompted Jarvis Cocker's stage invasion the following year.

Jackson had also married Elvis Presley's daughter, Lisa-Marie, in a match made in tabloid heaven. Having publicly admitted to painkiller addiction – used to cope with the abuse scandal – he was clearly an angry man on this single and album.

The 52-page booklet that came with *HIStory* contained messages of support from celebrities such as Elizabeth Taylor, a list of Jackson's many awards and pictures of the artist with four separate US presidents.

Like this single, *HIStory* was a commercial success, but many felt the double-album format of greatest hits/new material served only to highlight Jackson's creative stasis in the '90s, in contrast to his more productive years in the preceding two decades. Jackson collapsed during rehearsals in America; his recuperation from a viral infection coincided with the news that his marriage to Lisa-Marie was over.

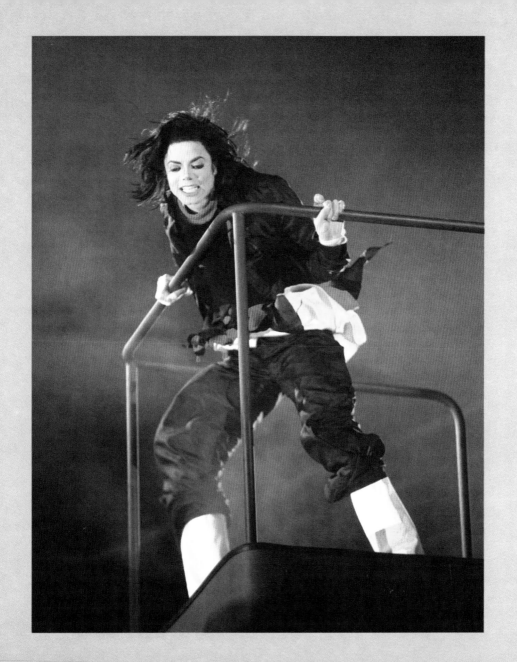

70 Can't Get You Out Of My Head
Kylie Minogue

Release Date: 29.09.01
No. Weeks In Chart: 25
Reached No. 1: 29.09.01
Total Sales: 1,037,235

Total global sales of this irresistible pop classic exceeded three million copies, and included Kylie's highest-ever chart placing in the US (at No. 7).

The diminutive Kylie is one of two actresses-turned-singers in this list from the Australian soap *Neighbours* (see also No. 85). She first won fame as Charlene, on-screen wife and off-screen lover of Jason Donovan.

After plunging into a pop career with the help of Pete Waterman, Kylie racked up thirteen straight Top Ten hits and four No. 1s. The sex-kitten pop image emerged when she started dating the late Michael Hutchence of INXS, although her chart career stalled somewhat during the early to mid-'90s. A faltering re-invention on the Deconstruction dance label seemed to suggest that Kylie's high-profile chart life was petering out.

A solid return to form was achieved with the million-selling *Light Years* album and then, in the summer of 2000, she released 'Spinning Around', a No. 1 smash that relaunched her career at the highest level overnight. Working with some of the industry's top songwriters, including former '90s pop starlet Cathy Dennis (who co-wrote this track), Kylie also delivered a five million-selling album, *Fever*, and a string of Top Ten hits. This award-winning single, affectionately known by many as the 'la la la song', was later melded with New Order's 'Blue Monday' (see No. 76) into a dance-floor hybrid classic. In 2001, Kylie's buttocks were heralded by the *Sun* newspaper as 'a national obsession'.

Kylie Minogue
Can't Get You Out Of My Head *(Parlophone)*

Exactly what you'd expect: slightly dated club sounds sculpted into something hard, sleek and seductive. All you can do is marvel at the machine-tooled efficiency of it all. The winner, then, of this week's Mildy Diverting Diva Of No Discernible Purpose award.

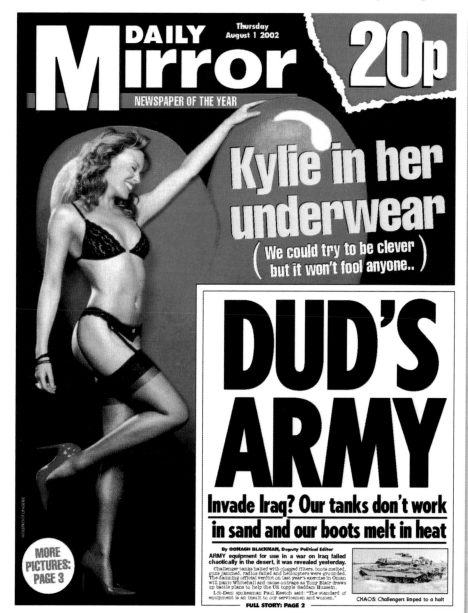

DAILY Mirror

NEWSPAPER OF THE YEAR

Thursday
August 1 2002

20p

Kylie in her underwear

(We could try to be clever
but it won't fool anyone..)

HOUSEHOLD LINGERIE

MORE
PICTURES:
PAGE 3

DUD'S ARMY

Invade Iraq? Our tanks don't work in sand and our boots melt in heat

By OONAGH BLACKMAN, Deputy Political Editor

ARMY equipment for use in a war on Iraq failed chaotically in the desert, it was revealed yesterday.

Challenger tanks halted with clogged filters, boots melted, guns jammed, radios failed and helicopters were grounded. The damning official verdict on last year's exercise in Oman will panic Whitehall and cause outrage as Tony Blair draws up battle plans to help the US topple Saddam Hussein.

Lib-Dem spokesman Paul Keetch said: "The standard of equipment is an insult to our servicemen and women."

FULL STORY: PAGE 2

CHAOS: Challengers limped to a halt

71 Blue (Da Ba Dee)
Eiffel 65

Release Date: 21.08.99
No. Weeks In Chart: 26
Reached No. 1: 25.09.99
Total Sales: 1,023,536

Rather oddly, the song was released to almost no fanfare and tiny sales, but over the summer months of 1999 copies started to fly out of the shops.

Not quite a one-hit wonder (its successor hit No. 3), this tune launched a fleeting visit to the charts by this Italian dance trio.

The group's name was generated at random by programmed software, but by mistake the band scribbled the digits '65' on the slip of paper that was then sent to the printing plant. Singer Jeffrey Jey, a Sicilian working and living in Turin, Italy, was a former accountancy student who hooked up with producer/musician Maurizio Lobina, also from Turin, and leading Italian DJ Gabry Ponte.

The lyrics, which are simply Jey's take on the colour that he feels best represents his daily life, repeat the word 'blue' no fewer than 27 times. Like the other Italian dance hits in the list – namely, Whigfield (see No. 64) and Black Box (see No. 94) – Eiffel 65 enjoyed almost total domination of the European and even South American dance charts, hitting No. 1 in the UK with just over one million sales (more than Oasis' 'Wonderwall'). At one point in 1999, the curiously entitled 'Blue (Da Ba Dee)' was being played on the radio every 150 seconds.

EIFFEL 65

BLUE

[DA BA DEE]

THE ORIGINAL ITALIAN MEGAHIT

72 Can We Fix It?
Bob The Builder

Release Date: 16.12.00
No. Weeks In Chart: 22
Reached No. 1: 23.12.00
Total Sales: 1,008,777

Within six months of the show first being screened, over £15 million of related merchandise had been sold.

Just as Oasis were plucked from the grim urban decay of Manchester's council estates and transformed into multi-millionaire rock gods, so Bob (a builder) and his cat, Pilchard, have found themselves similarly thrust into the media spotlight.

It all began in spring 1999, when the pair were approached by Hit Entertainment about filming a 'reality' TV show of their daily life – building things, fixing problems and generally having a good time. On the show's launch, Bob, his business partner Wendy, and their crew of fun-loving building machines – Scoop the digger, Muck the dump truck, Roley the steamroller, Lofty the crane and Dizzy the cement mixer – were taken aback by the public's feverish response.

Like so many other stars of soaps and reality shows, it was inevitable that a recording career was quickly mooted. Taking the theme tune from the show and mutating it with cunning garage beats and anthemic feel-good 'Yes we can!' vocals, Bob's debut single 'Can We Fix It?' was the huge million-selling Christmas hit of 2000. Sales were helped by his fur-lined Liam Gallagher-style jackets and rampant crowd-surfing, which were all captured on the promo video for the single. Even the previously all-conquering Westlife could not compete and were left trailing at No. 2. Bob's UK video release enjoyed double the sales of his debut single and a series of arena shows were sold out in a matter of hours.

Bob disproved the doubters who said he was a one-hit wonder by releasing a follow-up smash, 'Mambo No. 5', and a critically applauded multi-genre album (including Latino-infected pop, line-dancing classics and the haunting 'What Can I Be?', a moving duet with Spud the Scarecrow). Bob has since gone on to 'crack' America, selling three million videos and two million books in addition to millions of records – his world tour took in a hundred separate markets, all enjoying commercial success similar to this UK chart-topper.

In the US, the president and CEO of a global corporation even dressed up in overalls, red plaid shirts and hard hats to woo Bob and his chums to sign to their company. At the time of going to press, it was unclear if Bob was still in the studio writing his next album, or if he had gone home for tea with Wendy.

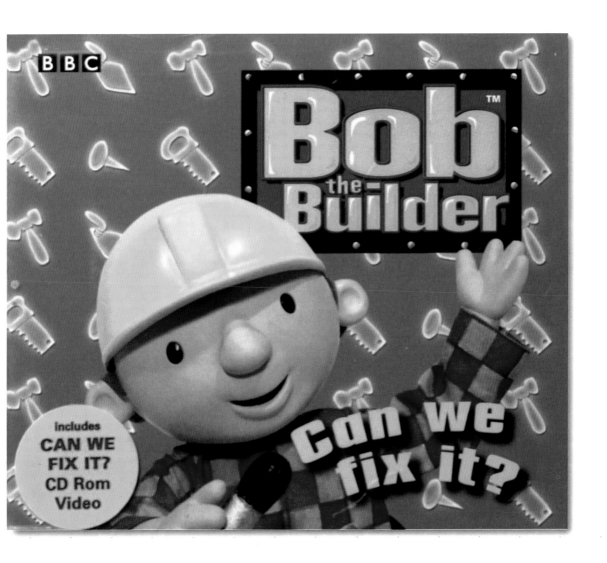

The '80s

Mainstream style now revolved around power dressing – Porsche-driving high-flyers with mobile phones, and women with 'big' hair, padded shoulders and sharp suits.

The decade brought us MTV, fashion magazines such as *The Face* and *i-D*, the Rubik's Cube, the Sony Walkman, home computers and video games. But the '80s were perhaps most sartorially memorable for the multitude of subcultural tribes that proliferated on the underground.

The clean lines and smart suits of Two Tone did not survive long into the '80s. Soon, the ludicrously clad New Romantics were swaying towards the top of the charts, bringing with them one of music's most over-dressed genres. Spandau Ballet seemed content with appearing on stage in a variety of rugs, while Duran Duran stole the hearts of a million teens with their frilly shirts and swashbuckling boots. However, it is perhaps Boy George who will be remembered as the fashion icon of the early '80s. His gender-bending look and lifestyle was a genuine one-off, although Marilyn Manson and Pete Burns were also tabloid regulars. Undeterred by the media heckling he received on a daily basis, his enigmatic dress sense secured him acres of tabloid coverage and, eventually, massive record sales (see No. 29).

Madonna's thrift-store gypsy chic, best seen in the 1985 movie *Desperately Seeking Susan*, was hugely popular and the heavy bangles,

7 June 1986　　　　50p　　　US $2.25 (by air)　　　　　　　　ISSN 0028 6362

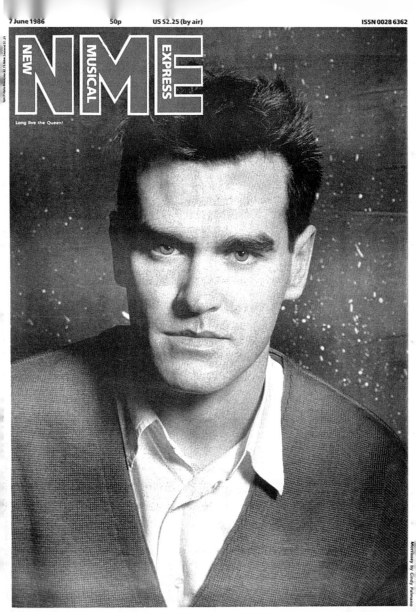

Long live the Queen!

gged skirts, fingerless gloves and
e of hair were her trademark. Such
in complete contrast to the previous
craze – the 'Frankie Says' black-and-
irt (see No.'s 7 and 22).

de also saw fleeting, but high-impact
Adam Ant's unique look was pure
t relied a little too heavily on Ant's
s (see No. 83). Turning up at the
 dressed as the local village's own
hwayman guaranteed any fledgling
more than a thump in the face.
it was a brave kid who copied Phil
p-sided haircut and make-up, which
Human League's profile (see No. 25).
ere also geographical pockets of
h the student icons The Smiths
om Manchester; ditto the flared
f the Stone Roses and the so-called
r baggy scene. Down in the West
the grebo was crawling out from
tone, sporting loud T-shirts, crimped
and cut-off shorts in support of
ly named bands such as Ned's Atomic
Pop Will Eat Itself and The Wonder
e south-east, the M25 cordoned off a
Essex as prime rave territory, taking
sed warehouses and agricultural
and filling them with whistle-
miley culture worshippers.

site ends to the champagne-swilling
rs, two subcultures epitomised the
 the '80s underground: the perpetual
the goth, and the cartoon
ce of psychobilly. Possibly the most
of all the subcultures, goths wear

anything as long as it is black.
faces and jet-black eye make-up,
'80s lived vicariously through
such as The Mission, Sisters of
Cure. Spawned in 1981 in th
named Batcave club in London,
pale-faced, doom-obsessed
gathered a large and cult follow

Psychobilly was hated by a
who wasn't involved in it, e
industry. Truly anti-establ
hardcore cult demanded a s
allegiance while offering a w
snakebite by the gallon a
soundtrack rooted in rockabilly
explosion giving England's you
rebel, the psychobilly phenomei
baton gallantly. Flying in the
rockabilly, it upset the purists
fashion stance. People crossed t
psychobilly approached: multi-
bleached jeans, DMs halfway u
a multitude of tattoos prevai
bands like The Stray Cats an
enjoyed chart success, whereas
far less commercial, far more p

The first true psychobilly
Meteors: Often covered in fake b
the pioneers of the movement.
mecca was the Klubfoot at th
Hammersmith, west London. Th
spread, and for a while it see
teenager on the underground
tattoo. Not the sort of person
toothed and skimpy short-weari
would have enjoyed meeting in

U2 in Japan, part 2 ★ THE WONDER STUFF
PIXIES ★ JUNGLE BROTHERS ★ CHRISTIANS
JIVE BUNNY ★ ANTOINE de *Rapido*

IS THIS THE REEL LIFE?

NME

On The Piste

BLIND DATE
Moz, Axl,
Tanita
and Matt
get matched
(sort of)

**IAN McCULLOCH
FUZZBOX
JOHN PEEL
TRACY TRACY**
flesh out their
film fantasies

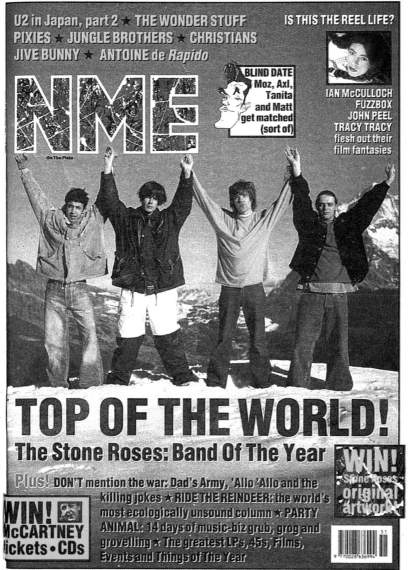

TOP OF THE WORLD!
The Stone Roses: Band Of The Year

WIN!
Stone Roses
original
artwork

Plus! DON'T mention the war: Dad's Army, 'Allo 'Allo and the
killing jokes ★ RIDE THE REINDEER: the world's
most ecologically unsound column ★ PARTY
ANIMAL: 14 days of music-biz grub, grog and
grovelling ★ The greatest LPs, 45s, Films,
Events and Things of The Year

WIN!
McCARTNEY
tickets • CDs

9 770025 636994

The Stone Roses photographed by Tim Jarvis

73 Merry Christmas Everybody
Slade

Release Date: 15.12.73
No. Weeks In Chart: 34
Reached No. 1: 15.12.73
Total Sales: 1,006,500

The fertile writing partnership between Noddy Holder and Jim Lea produced this, their sixth and final chart-topper.

One of several festive hits in this list to have benefited from repeated Yuletide sales, this Christmas staple should keep Noddy Holder and crew in platform shoes well into old age.

Initially a long-haired reggae and soul backing band, Slade mutated into the first skinhead band before becoming glam rock's premier exponents. The skinhead's short trousers were (mis)appropriated and complemented with outlandish platforms, lurid glam clothing and some of the worst mullets in rock, to create a formula that turned Slade into one of the biggest acts of the decade.

The fertile writing partnership between Holder and Jim Lea made them the first band to have three singles enter straight in at No. 1 – this track was their sixth and final chart-topper, one of only a handful not to use colloquial Black Country spelling, and the first Christmas-themed No. 1 since Harry Belafonte's Yuletide classic, 'Mary's Boy Child' (see No. 51).

Legend has it that Lea was struck by the idea for the tune while in a shower in Memphis, Tennessee, and scribbled it down on a scrap of sopping-wet paper while wrapped only in a towel. On the single's release in 1973, Slade

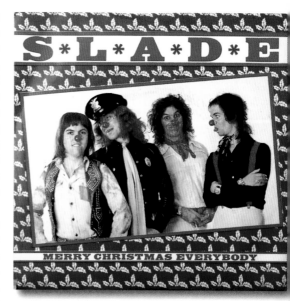

succeeded in shifting 250,000 copies in one day, then 450,000 in six months.

Since then, thousands of yearly sales have seen several chart re-entries (seven in the '80s alone) and succeeded in pushing this single past the million-copies-sold mark. Given the trend, it seems likely that the figure will rise.

THERE IS ONLY ONE
SLADE

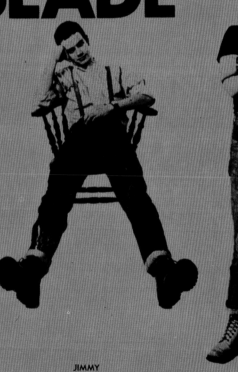

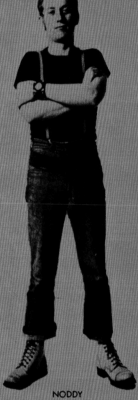

DON   DAVE   JIMMY   NODDY

74 Save Your Kisses For Me
Brotherhood Of Man

Release Date: 13.03.76
No. Weeks In Chart: 16
Reached No. 1: 27.03.76
Total Sales: 1,006,200

Brotherhood Of Man were seen by many people as Britain's answer to Abba. It was ironic, therefore, that their greatest hit was replaced at the top after six weeks by the Swedish foursome's 'Fernando'.

Although they will be forever associated with this 1976 Eurovision Song Contest winner, Brotherhood of Man had existed in some form or other since the late '60s. Producer and composer Tony Hiller worked under the group's name with a variety of seasoned session singers – notably a pre-fame Elton John, who once backed them on an edition of *Top of the Pops*.

Brotherhood Of Man's debut single, 'United We Stand', had become something of a signature tune for the rising gay liberation movement in America, released as it was in 1970, just one year after the Stonewall riots. However, it was 'Save Your Kisses For Me' that indelibly marked the group's place in pop history. Brotherhood of Man went to the Eurovision final in The Hague and won with this immensely catchy pop-ditty accompanied by simple dance steps – a musical innocence that was staring down the barrel of soon-to-explode punk.

An impressive 164 points secured Brotherhood of Man their Eurovision victory, and the accompanying television coverage helped the single to sell a shade over one million copies.

The tune also became the first UK Eurovision entry to climb into the US Top 40, although it was to mark the peak of the group's chart action on that side of the Atlantic.

The track hit the top spot in 34 countries and was one of the Top Ten selling singles of the '70s. Perhaps surprisingly, it remains the best-selling Eurovision song ever, ahead even of Abba's classic 'Waterloo'.

The group enjoyed two further No. 1 records in under two years before their chart career drew to a close. They still perform regularly on the gay cabaret circuit and at holiday camps.

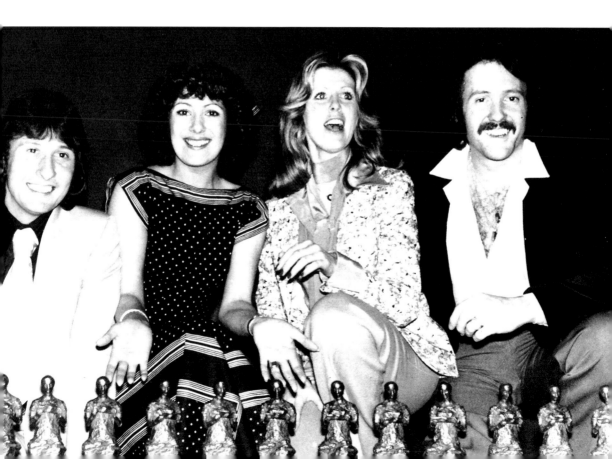

75 Eye Level
Simon Park Orchestra

Release Date: 25.11.72
No. Weeks In Chart: 24
Reached No. 1: 29.09.73
Total Sales: 1,005,500

This strident instrumental arrangement was initially released in November 1972 to coincide with the first screening of the TV series *Van Der Valk*.

The only appearance in the charts by the Simon Park Orchestra, this instrumental song was a huge success, fuelled by the popularity of the television police show *Van Der Valk*, for which it was the theme tune.

Simon Park had studied for a music degree at Oxford University before working at De Wolfe Music Publishers, specialists in film and television scores. He was given snippets of this tune, probably based on an old Dutch folk tune of uncertain origin, by a composer from the Netherlands. His arrangement was released in November 1972 to coincide with the first series of *Van Der Valk*, but only reached No. 41.

The show was based on the Nicholas Freeling novels and featured the late Barry Foster, an actor whose distinctive blond locks and sullen personality regularly drew audiences of up to eight million. With little or no marketing, the second series helped lift the theme tune to the No. 1 spot eight months after its initial release, where it remained for one month. Its reign at the top spot was ended only by the teen heartthrob David Cassidy.

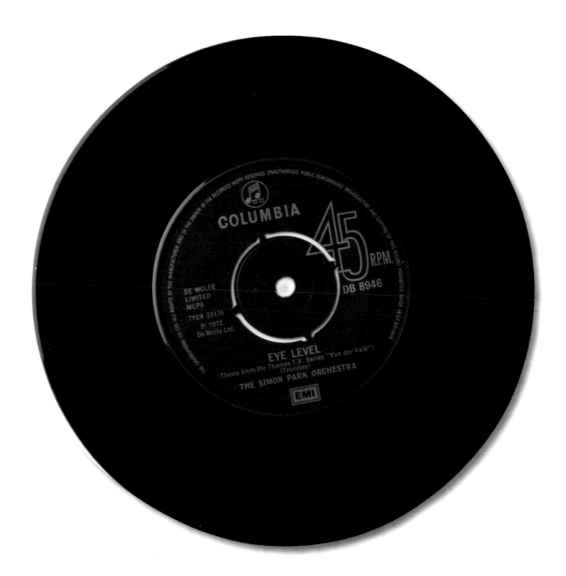

76 Blue Monday
New Order

Release Date: 19.03.83
No. Weeks In Chart: 53
Reached No. 1: N/A
Total Sales: 1,001,400

This record is one of the most influential and pivotal dance records ever released and the biggest-selling twelve-inch of all time – yet it never reached No. 1.

'Blue Monday' is thought to be the result of combined studio experiments with LSD and a new drum machine. Spearheaded by Hook's trademark bass lines, Sumner's atonal vocalisation of his rather abstract lyrics and the spine-tingling keyboards, this track became an instant classic. The track '586' on the watershed album *Power, Corruption & Lies* is seen as a precursor to 'Blue Monday', which did not originally feature on that acclaimed long player.

Initially released only as a twelve-inch, a multitude of remixes and different formats have created a mini-collector's market – only 25 copies of one particular seven-inch edit were pressed, of which bassist Peter Hook claims to have a stack in his closet.

The song spent almost a year in the chart, and remains the biggest-selling twelve-inch ever released in the UK – and this, despite the fact that initially, it rose no higher than No. 12 in the charts.

When first released with a secret, colour-coded sleeve, the half a million copies sold did not earn Factory Records a Gold disc as they were not members of the BPI (British Phonographic Industry). Instead, Factory Records guru Tony Wilson had some gold statuettes made up.

This track sealed New Order's brave new incarnation from the embers of Joy Division and single-handedly reinvented dance music – it has since been credited with spawning techno and blurring the lines between a host of previously distinct genres.

Legend has it that German electro-pop pioneers Kraftwerk were so in awe of this song that they insisted on renting the same studio as the one New Order used.

Initial sales have been supplemented by remixes in both 1988 and 1995, almost continual references in the music media and even its use on a cunningly amalgamated remix of Kylie Minogue's 'Can't Get You Out of My Head' (see No. 70).

And in case you were wondering, the New Order song has no relation to the Fats Domino song of the same name.

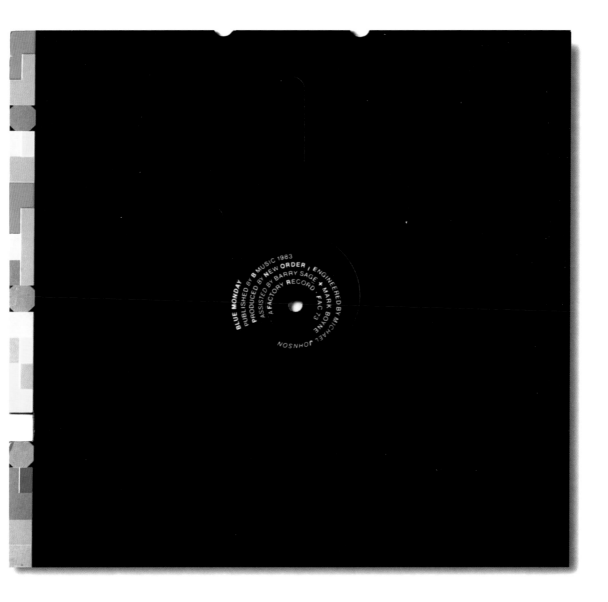

77

Long Haired Lover From Liverpool
Little Jimmy Osmond

Release Date:	25.11.72
No. Weeks In Chart:	27
Reached No. 1:	23.12.72
Total Sales:	998,000

The pre-teen Jimmy would regularly sing in front of thousands of people, only to be scolded later by his luxury hotel manager for playing with toys in the corridor.

Replacing 'My Ding-a-Ling' by Chuck Berry, some 37 years his senior, this solo hit for the youngest of the entertainment family The Osmonds is the biggest-selling song to fall just short of one million sales (998,000). Jimmy made his debut aged only three in a Las Vegas showroom, where he would do Sinatra and Elvis impressions – one night, Sinatra watched him from the side of the stage and later gave him his trademark hat.

Jimmy's popularity in the UK surpassed that in his native America, as indeed it did for the rest of The Osmonds, devout Mormons from Salt Lake City who had originally formed a barber-shop quartet. Seen as rivals to the Jackson Five, Osmond-mania was a bona fide teen-pop sensation in the early '70s. Although most pubescent emotions were focussed on the older pin-up looks of Donny, rather than on the somewhat chubby younger sibling, Jimmy enjoyed his own solo success with this song (although he admitted he didn't know where Liverpool was). A tribute song, 'Little Jimmy', was released at this time by then Rhodesian singer Gwynneth Joubert.

Jimmy later became a successful businessman and promoter, and now regularly performs at the Osmond Family Theatre in Missouri.

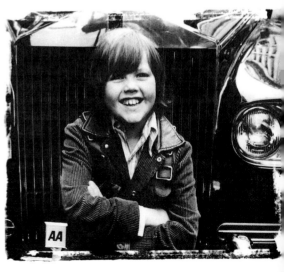

BATTLE OF THE BOPPERS

The day the Osmonds and the Jacksons flew in

CALL IT GOOD timing or bad management: the two biggest of the screamy bands, the Osmonds and the Jackson Five, both arrived within three hours of each other at London Airport on Sunday. Both are staying at the same hotel in London — and on November 13, both return to America.

I trust that the airport's security will be out in greater force by then than it was on Sunday when — at only 6.20 a.m. — hundreds of weenyboppers and teenyboppers were out in force at Terminal 3 for a glimpse, scream or touch with the J.5.

Around 7 a.m. the screaming, leaping and yelling began in earnest ... and this just at the photographers, one of whom had announced "don't worry, they'll be here in 10 minutes."

When the Jackson Five did arrive, their black, smiling but tired faces pushing through the door past customs, all hell broke loose. It was mass pushing, screaming, crying and crush.

Two of the J.5 fell down. One was separated from the main group and Randy and Michael both cried, so overcome with emotion ("Not fear", they told me later).

The police tried in vain to control the crowd. Photographer Robert Ellis lost £100 worth of lens in the crush and within two minutes the whole band had been pushed into a waiting car.

Now the car ... that's another thing. Around £500 of damage they reckon — all done in the space of about 30 seconds. It had scratches, dents, the lot.

Still at the airport, many of the girls cried — one said: "I touched him," and burst into tears realising she'd actually touched Michael Jackson. Some of them tried to run after the car on its way to London.

Others surveyed their ripped jackets and scuffed shoes — while less fortunate ones were left cried with cuts and bruises.

But the resilience was there,

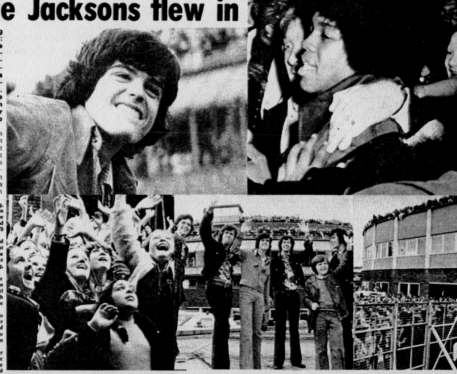

A hand appeared around a curtain. And a thousand girls screamed.

inconspicuous despite the word DONNY embroidered over their trousers or jackets or clutching a picture of Michael from a maga-

crowd at the other side looking for Donny — rushed over too.

"Well the Jackson Five are

trying to keep the crowd from breaking in. And at a side door I'm offered £1.50 to open the door to let some of them in.

jobsworth employed by the hotel, getting pushed and shoved in an effort to keep "them", as he described the crowd, out of the

with. There was no escape.

The national Press was astounded although it would be easy, but naive, to regard the whole

78 Another Brick In The Wall (Part 2)
Pink Floyd

Release Date: 1.12.79
No. Weeks In Chart: 12
Reached No. 1: 15.12.79
Total Sales: 995,000

A bleak, Orwellian vision that was a surprising pop hit – Pink Floyd were still working on this pivotal single two weeks before its release date.

By the late '70s, punk had blown away the cobwebs of Prog Rock and Two Tone was already festering in Coventry's side-streets. Yet Pink Floyd still secured their first and only UK and US No. 1 single with this track.

The famous schoolchildren's chant was a recording of pupils at Islington Green School, London, captured on tape by a producer – the band were tax exiles and therefore unable to enter the UK. The accompanying video, featuring cartoonist Gerald Scarfe's animated and darkly sinister teacher-hammers and children being pushed through a meat mincer, secured acres of TV coverage.

Although this was the first No. 1 single of the '80s, it was only the third-biggest single of that year, behind Blondie and Art Garfunkel (see No.'s 50 and 53). Roger Waters later recorded a version of this track with the Bleeding Heart Band and Cyndi Lauper.

The song was taken from the album *The Wall*, which is regarded by many as the greatest concept record of all time – allegedly inspired by an incident whereby Waters spat at an irritating and noisy fan at a Montreal concert. Record company files reveal that this album took 1,279 hours to record.

The staggeringly expensive live show for this project – including 45 tons of props – was performed only 29 times and at a financial loss (Waters never played with the Floyd again on stage, and left the band in 1984). The Alan Parker-directed movie of the album, starring Bob Geldof in the lead role of Pink, was released in 1982. In 1990, Waters performed *The Wall* stage show as a free concert in front of over 400,000 people in Berlin.

Pink Floyd have enjoyed only two other Top 20 hits – rather surprising for a band who, in 1990, were supported on stage at Knebworth by such pop luminaries as Paul McCartney, Eric Clapton, Elton John, Cliff Richard, Phil Collins, Mark Knopfler and Led Zeppelin's Robert Plant and Jimmy Page.

Although described as an 'album band', it is worth noting that neither Pink Floyd's *The Wall* nor *Dark Side of the Moon* hit the No. 1 position in the album charts.

**PINK FLOYD: Another Brick In
The Wall, Pt.II (Harvest)**.

For the Floyd, Christmas
product comes in larger
diameters, this year two of
'em; the prime function of
'Another Brick, Pt.II' is as a
taster for the bigger stuff. And
as such, it's fairly cunningly
conceived, complete with
easily-memorable
moron-choir parts, simple
enough for the thickest of
terrace terrorists. Expect to
hear it accompanying the
sound of bladders (human or
swine) being kicked around on
Saturday afternoons.

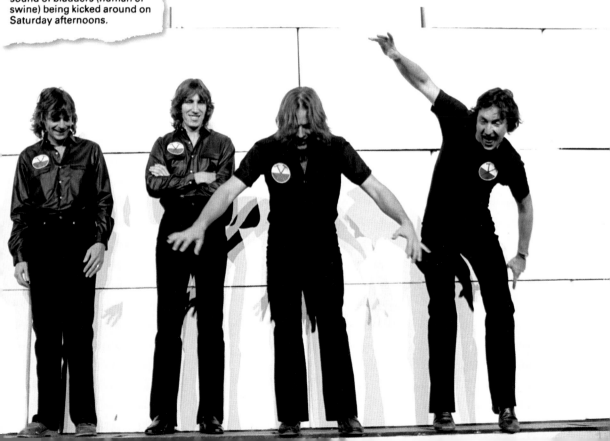

The
Rave
Scene

r decades now, music and youth subculture have been
extricably linked, close partners in crime, as it were,
ce the advent of rock 'n' roll.

ough many of the mega-star names in
book can hardly be described as
cultural', there has always been a
ving undercurrent of alternative music
fashion on the underbelly of music's
t behemoths.

er the years, these changing tides in
ultural development have taken on many
ly defined characteristics. By highlighting
one such development – the rave scene of

the late '80s – it is possible to identify many of
the defining criteria.

During the summer of 1988, a new musical
form began sweeping through the UK's
clubland, with its hypnotic beats and new-age
drug culture – Acid House. The origin of the
term is unclear, although many people claim it
was inspired by the group Phuture's 'Acid Trax'
single of 1987. The musical roots of the form
are equally difficult to identify. Many saw it as

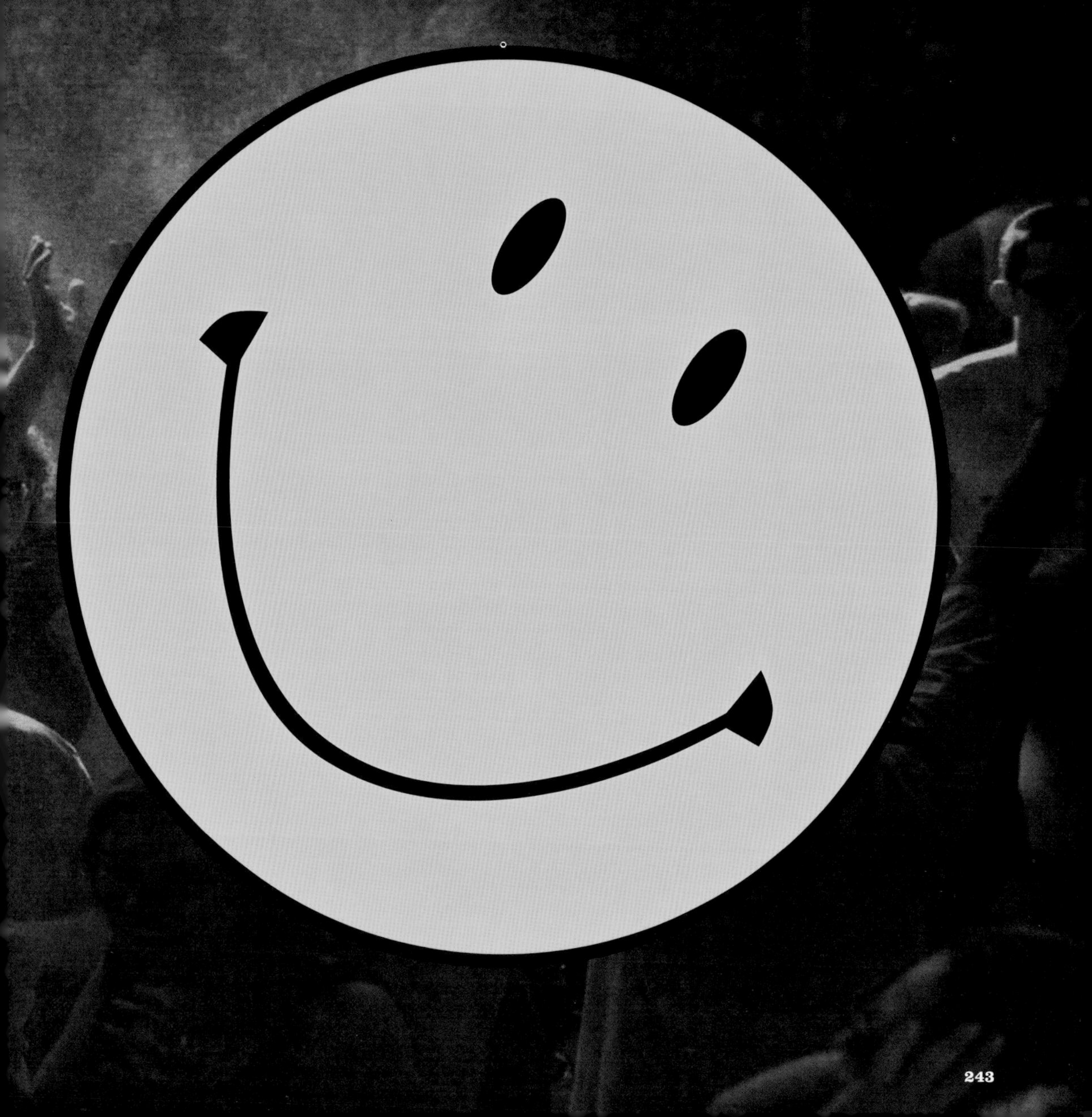

evolving from the musical mecca of Chicago. Others said it hailed from Detroit, and laid the credit at the feet of people such as Juan Atkins, Derrick May, Kevin Saunderson and other innovative DJs and musicians.

Whatever its actual origins, the new, minimalist Acid House had many musical cousins; yet its mind-altering frequencies, relentless rhythms, unconventional structures and off-beat soundscapes imbued it with a weirdness and unorthodoxy all of its own. While house music tempered its rhythmic obsession by incorporating more melodies and harmonies, Acid House pursued rhythm to new extremes, using the technology that had broken the mould of traditional live, instrumental music – in the process producing beats that could never be simulated by flesh-and-blood musicians.

The music soon crossed the Atlantic from the US to the UK, although some report ecstasy in Ibiza as far back as 1984, and clubs such as Shoom and Project Club were the real innovators on these shores. The scene was introduced to Britain through massive, illegal warehouse parties: rave had arrived.

With the so-called smart bars selling high-energy, strictly non-alcoholic, caffeine-pumped drinks to fuel the marathon dancing sessions, the culture rapidly adopted a recycled hippie mantra, and its 'love vibe' and benign communality created what came to be known as the 'Second Summer Of Love'.

The media did not like it one bit (*Top of the Pops* even banned some 'acid' tracks), nor did the authorities and the older generation. But this attempted criminalisation served only to heighten the rebellious flavour – and thus the popularity – of the massive all-night parties. Ironically, many of the people who were now condemning rave as barbaric, mindless, repetitive and nihilistic were those very same people who had grown up in the '60s, when the same criticisms were being levelled at their own amphetamine stutter of 'My Generation'.

The mainstream snub of the 'Smiley culture' would take on a more determined edge in October 1989, when special anti-drug squads were set up to combat the spreading phenomenon; but for now, the baggy jeans, long hair, psychedelic patterns and loose clothes of the 'ravers' roamed free across the country. Pirate radio stations filtered new material out from under the noses of the media, and the sheer scale of some all-nighters (frequently running to tens of thousands of ravers) meant that the authorities seemingly had little power to stop them.

The scene was most prevalent in the south-east of England; here, the M25 motorway became celebrated on thousands of flyers for illegal parties, since it cut off a neat section of south-western Essex, which then became a haven for the phenomenon.

The early raves were secretive affairs, with people being given phone numbers to call or meetings to attend at service stations along the M25, whereupon they could find out the clandestine location of that night's party. The dearth of accurate media documentation further heightened the sense that this was utterly, an underground experience.

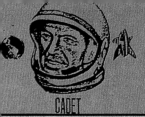

● Balearic Beat may have been last year's thing but Ibiza still has a direct line to the UK club scene. RICHARD NOISE survives a week of the tack and the sleaze, the agony and the ecstasy, to discover 'the greatest club in the world'...

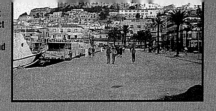

E VIVA AMNESIA

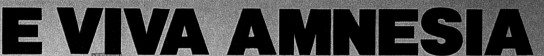

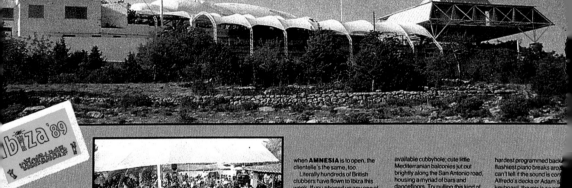

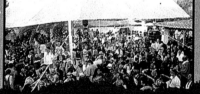

Ibiza! Costa del t package

when **AMNESIA** is to open, the clientelle's the same, too.

Literally hundreds of British clubbers have flown to Ibiza this week. If you phoned up any one of the countless travel agents that litter the London listings mags in the week proceeding Amnesia's opening, you'd get the same story – "Don't ask me for tickets to Ibiza –

available cubbyhole; cute little Mediterranean balconies jut out brightly along the San Antonio road, housing a myriad of bars and dancefloors. Try pulling this kind of trick in Bradford.

Just like in the Wham! song, all the drinks are free, only these come in a form of punch apparently laced with ecstasy and mescalin. And I'm su

hardest programmed back flashiest piano breaks aro can't tell if the sound is co Alfredo's decks or Adam's keyboard, the mix is so go him here when you can.

As the sun rose over A open roof, the British co were at a loss for words of the Hill Street Blues th

Then, just as rave seemed to be at its best, the beast of commerciality smothered it. High-street stores were selling Smiley logos on T-shirts and bags, Euro-pop versions of the rave theme were belittling the originals and, worst of all, there was kindergarten rave. Dozens of so-called kiddy samples, taken from

children's television shows or adverts, were spliced into a stereotypical acid beat and were usually guaranteed sound chart success Tracks such as Shaft's 'Roobarb and Custard' Urban Hype's 'Trip to Trumpton', and the Smarties' 'Sesame's Treet' had all done little to stabilise rave's dwindling credibility

The Prodigy were accused of opening the floodgates for the death of rave with their No. 3 single, 'Charly', which took its central sample from a children's information broadcast of the '70s. Prodigy were perhaps the most recognisable group in a genre that was often largely faceless. They have since gone on to break free of their rave origins to become the world's biggest-selling hard dance act.

At the time, however, they were unjustly accused. There was no mention of the responsibility for rave's decline being borne by the scene's own greed – or rather the outsiders who siphoned off the financial rewards. There was no mention either of the growing adulteration of ecstasy with amphetamines and dangerously impure additives, which suddenly plunged anyone 'indulging' at a party into a narcotic round of Russian Roulette.

There was no mention of the snob DJs who insisted on playing only the rarest and most obscure of of tracks in the petty battle for dance-floor kudos, nor of the concerted mainstream media policy of besmirching rave and its followers. No mention either of the contextual truth – in other words, the fact that 'Charly' came eighteen months before many of these poor imitations finally decided to make their dash for cash.

Rave was arguably the most powerful youth movement for a decade, perhaps the first time since punk that parents had been petrified over where their children were, and yet it degenerated into novelty cartoon samples. That said, it boasted many of the classic elements of a genuine subcultural movement: the uncertain origins, the stench of the underground and the non-establishment; the absolute rebelliousness; the authorities' moves to outlaw or at least stifle it and the resulting extra cachet it enjoyed as a contraband lifestyle; the disdain and lack of co-operation of the bemused musical establishment; the musical splintering into a myriad of offshoots; then the slow but relentless insemination of the mainstream eventually taking over music and fashion as just another corporate means to an end. Then at last, the final death throes – in the form of self-parody, as prime-time pop shows featured gas-mask-wearing white-jumpsuited ravers long after this was even vaguely relevant to the scene at grass-roots level.

Without the mainstream superstars, the underground would have nothing to grind against. Although rave finds no place in this Top 100 singles of all time, it is a superlative example of a subculture that represents the very opposite of the super-commerciality that such a list heralds.

So rave on, Sir Cliff.

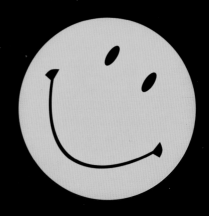

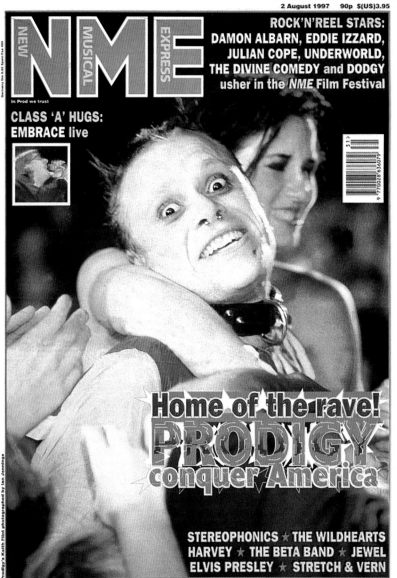

2 August 1997   90p $(US)3.95

NME
NEW MUSICAL EXPRESS

In Prod we trust

ROCK'N'REEL STARS:
DAMON ALBARN, EDDIE IZZARD,
JULIAN COPE, UNDERWORLD,
THE DIVINE COMEDY and DODGY
usher in the *NME* Film Festival

CLASS 'A' HUGS:
EMBRACE live

Germany Dm 8.50 Spain/Fax N50

Prodigy's Keith Flint photographed by Ian Jennings

Home of the rave!
PRODIGY
conquer America

STEREOPHONICS ★ THE WILDHEARTS
HARVEY ★ THE BETA BAND ★ JEWEL
ELVIS PRESLEY ★ STRETCH & VERN

79 Don't Cry For Me Argentina
Julie Covington

Release Date: 25.12.76
No. Weeks In Chart: 18
Reached No. 1: 12.02.77
Total Sales: 993,000

Covington sang on the studio version of *Evita*, the musical, a full two years before its stage debut.

This actress and singer first found fame in the 1977 TV show *Rock Follies*, alongside Rula Lenska and Charlotte Cornwell, which resulted in the Top Ten single 'OK?'. But today she is best remembered for this plaintive song from one of the most popular musicals of the '70s.

Covington's performance in *Rock Follies* landed her the part of Eva Peron in Andrew Lloyd Webber and Tim Rice's *Evita*. This musical marked the pair's first work together since the *Jesus Christ Superstar* feature film. Peron had been the wife of Argentine president Juan Peron and had become something of a folklore legend in Argentina following her death in 1952 at the age of 33, and scenes of hysterical mourning accompanied her funeral.

Covington sang on the original concept album of the musical which, when it made its stage debut two years later, starred Elaine Page in the lead role opposite David Essex.

In more recent years, Peron's role has been made famous once more by Madonna, who starred in Alan Parker's film version of *Evita*. Madonna also enjoyed a Top Five hit with this same song in late 1996.

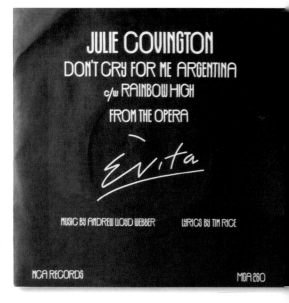

'Don't Cry For Me Argentina' was an international chart-topper, though it was to be Julie Covington's only No. 1 – a year later, she hit the Top 20 with a version of Alice Cooper's 'Only Women Bleed' and went on to work with Kate Bush, but shunned the spotlight and has since kept a relatively low profile.

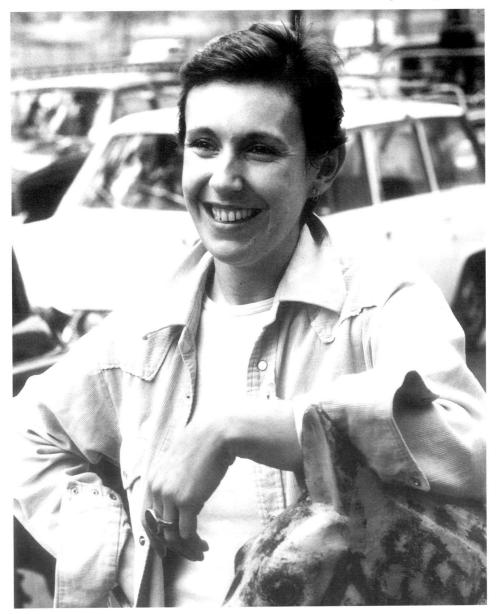

80 Eye Of The Tiger
Survivor

Release Date: 31.07.82
No. Weeks In Chart: 15
Reached No. 1: 4.09.82
Total Sales: 990,000

This Grammy-winning, Oscar-nominated feel-good track gave AOR rock group Survivor a transatlantic No. 1. The anthemic track has been used ever since for a million gym workouts and training sessions.

Written specifically for the film *Rocky III* – the third instalment of Sylvester Stallone's self-directed boxing chronicle – 'Eye of the Tiger' was the biggest of Survivor's two UK chart hits, and is one of the most instantly recognisable film themes of the '80s.

Although founder member Jim Peterik had enjoyed US hits with his group Ides of March, Survivor struggled to hit the big time until they soundtracked the gritty rags-to-riches tale of 'The Italian Stallion', boxer Rocky Bilboa – played by Sly himself.

Stallone was already a fan of Survivor's second album, *Premonition*, and asked the group to contribute to the soundtrack of his latest Rocky movie.

The first Rocky film, made in 1976, proved to be Stallone's breakthrough into the film world. It had a paltry budget of $1 million, was filmed in a record 28 days and grossed . . . well over $100 million. By the time *Rocky III* was being produced, it was one of the biggest-grossing film franchises of all time.

Survivor's song opened with a bombastic but catchy guitar riff and a thunderous beat – the two combining to create the aural equivalent of a boxer's punches. (The track took its title from the phrase used by Rocky's trainer Mickey to describe the pugilistic killer instinct.)

The single made Survivor the first US rock band in six years to have a UK No. 1, although the album of the same name stalled at No. 12. Stateside, the track spent six weeks at the top of the *Billboard* Hot 100, and the album became a million-seller.

'Burning Heart', from the *Rocky IV* film soundtrack, hit No. 5 in 1986, but thereafter Survivor never troubled the UK chart again. The band split in 1989, although a new Survivor arose in 1997.

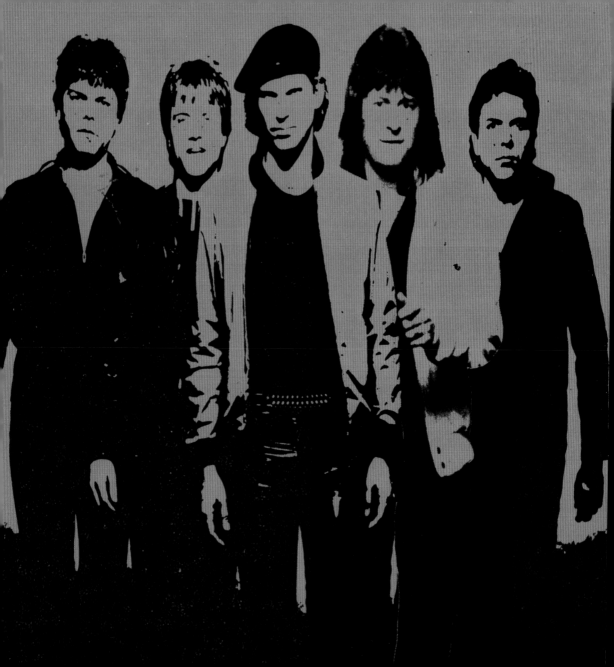

81 I'd Like To Teach The World To Sing
New Seekers

Release Date: 18.12.71
No. Weeks In Chart: 21
Reached No. 1: 8.01.72
Total Sales: 990,000

With this single, the New Seekers proudly boasted of knocking Benny Hill's hit 'Ernie' off No. 1 – only to be replaced by a somewhat more prestigious track, 'Telegram Sam', by T Rex.

After the split of The Seekers (see No. 30), Keith Potger formed the New Seekers, who will forever be associated with this Coca-Cola-related song. Potger initially performed with the group, but then moved behind the scenes to manage them.

Surpassing The Seekers' chart success, it was the use of this song for a Coca-Cola advert in 1972, complete with massed ranks of the world's (largely barefooted) peoples singing atop a mountain, that brought them their biggest hit. Initially, the song was just the advert's jingle; it was only released after huge public demand had swamped radio stations running the ad.

Lyrics were re-worded to remove any references to Coca-Cola – oddly, a version by The Hillside Singers was released first, but this was eclipsed by the New Seekers' definitive rendition. Their next hit was the 1972 Eurovision entry entitled 'Beg, Steal or Borrow', which fortunately did not score 'nil points'. A more rock-oriented image failed to halt their slide down the charts. In the '90s, the original line-up reformed for a millennium tour.

New Seekers
I'd Like To Teach The World To Sing (Polydor).

A FTER THEIR no. 1 hit, it was a surprise when the New Seekers failed to make the chart with their last single, " Old Fashioned Music." But I think this new one will rectify the omission, because it has everything going for it.

Originally this was the featured song in a Coca-Cola TV commercial in the States. —and I've recently noticed that they are now screening it in this country, too.

Immensely catchy, with an appealing lyric and bouncy beat, it makes an ideal show-case for the quintet's distinctive vocal blend and harmonies. The Seekers have a lot of TV coverage lined up, and with the Coke ad also working for them they're assured of mass exposure. But the key factor is that it's a catchy song, and the only thing that could prevent it from being a hit is over-saturation!

Tipped for the Charts

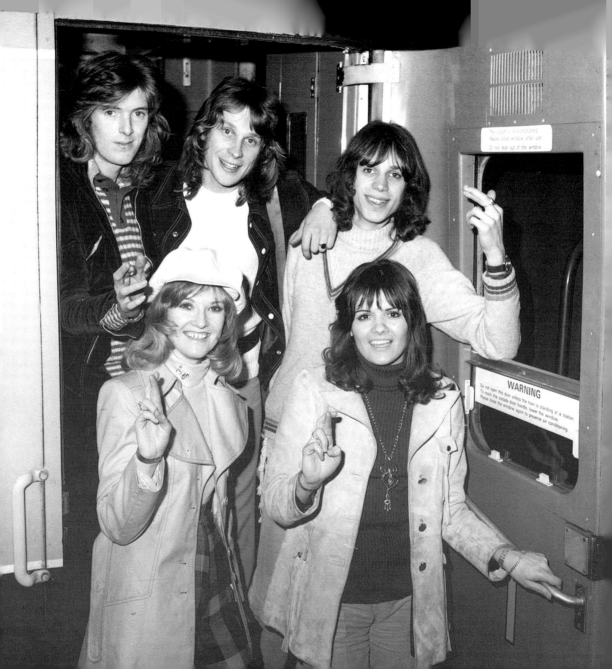

82 Tie A Yellow Ribbon Round The Ole Oak Tree
Dawn (featuring Tony Orlando)

Release Date: 10.03.73
No. Weeks In Chart: 40
Reached No. 1: 21.04.73
Total Sales: 988,000

With more than a thousand cover versions, this has since become a symbolic song for missing loved ones.

One of the most covered singles of all time, 'Tie A Yellow Ribbon' was reputedly inspired by the tale of an ex-convict returning home to his sweetheart in White Oak, Georgia, USA. The yellow ribbon was her sign to him that she still loved him – songwriters Irwin Levine and L Russell Brown caught this touching story on the newswire and immediately penned the tune. An alternative folklore theory has the love anecdote dating back to the American Civil War.

The band Dawn was actually fronted by Tony Orlando, a New York music manager and singer of several solo hits in the '60s who, initially, only agreed to sing the tune provided that he could remain anonymous in what was primarily a studio band. Indeed, Orlando didn't meet Dawn's two female singers, Hopkins and Wilson, until their second single, 'Knock Three Times', which was also a UK No.1 (again themed around the 'loves-me, loves-me-not' dilemma). Even bigger US success made Dawn a huge pop act. Their first live gig was at New York's Carnegie Hall after they had already sold nine million records – and six million since. *NME* voted them 1973's 'Number One Vocal Group in Europe'.

Huge commercial success and even their own television variety show did not dissuade Orlando from announcing his retirement, without prior warning to his band colleagues, live on stage in 1977. 'Tie A Yellow Ribbon' was re-released in America to celebrate the return of the Iran hostages in 1981.

BRITISH SINGLES

[Tuesday, 24th April, 1973]

1	1	TIE A YELLOW RIBBON Dawn (Bell)	6	1
3	2	HELLO! HELLO! I'M BACK AGAIN Gary Glitter (Bell)	4	2
2	3	GET DOWN Gilbert O'Sullivan (MAM)	7	3
4	4	I'M A CLOWN/SOME KIND OF A SUMMER David Cassidy (Bell)	6	3
10	5	DRIVE-IN SATURDAY David Bowie (RCA)	3	5
5	6	TWEEDLE DEE Jimmy Osmond (MGM)	5	5
6	7	PYJAMARAMA Roxy Music (Island)	7	6
7	8	LOVE TRAIN O'Jays (CBS)	7	7
12	9	ALL BECAUSE OF YOU Geordie (EMI)	4	9
9	10	NEVER NEVER NEVER Shirley Bassey (United Artists)	7	8
14	11	MY LOVE		

83 Stand and Deliver
Adam and The Ants

Release Date: 9.05.81
No. Weeks In Chart: 15
Reached No. 1: 9.05.81
Total Sales: 985,000

With his model good looks, unique blend of Native American and pirate style and twin drummers behind him, Adam Ant was the pop pin-up of the year.

The year 1981 was the year of the Ant. So-called 'Antmusic', named to avoid press pigeon-holing, was the phenomenon of 1981. Adam and the Ants notched up six hit singles during that year, even against stiff competition from Shakin' Stevens, one of the decade's biggest hit-makers. 'Stand and Deliver' entered the charts at No. 1 (the first of two chart-toppers that year, 'Prince Charming' being the other), displacing the skirt-snatching Eurovision pop of Bucks Fizz's 'Making Your Mind Up'. It stayed there for a month.

The grandson of a pure gypsy, Ant's early life was one of relative poverty; by his early twenties he was anorexic. A punk veteran, Ant (a.k.a. Stuart Goddard) had enjoyed little success in early bands Bazooka Joe and The B-Sides. It wasn't until Goddard adopted the persona of Adam Ant (he figured that if the insect-related pun of 'Beatles' had worked for the Fab Four. . .) that things really started to happen for him. Egged on by an image consultancy courtesy of Malcolm McLaren – for a £1,000 fee – Ant set about creating a new look and sound, although an early album, *Dirk Wears White Sox*, met with muted critical response. And when McLaren later stripped Ant of his backing band in order to form the press darlings Bow Wow Wow, the future was looking bleak for Antmusic.

However, with the recruitment of long-term writing partner Marco Pirroni (who had once appeared as part of an early incarnation of Siouxsie and the Banshees), two drummers and a large helping of African Burundi rhythms, Ant created a hugely popular formula, best heard on the top-selling album of the year, *Prince Charming*.

His accompanying videos became *Top of the Pops* staples. The promo for 'Stand and Deliver', complete with Ant's dandy highwayman character, was a classic pop moment of the '80s. Dissolving the group in 1982, Ant enjoyed a further UK No. 1 hit with 'Goody Two Shoes', before moving to the US to pursue an acting career. In 2002, he was charged with possession of an imitation firearm and assault.

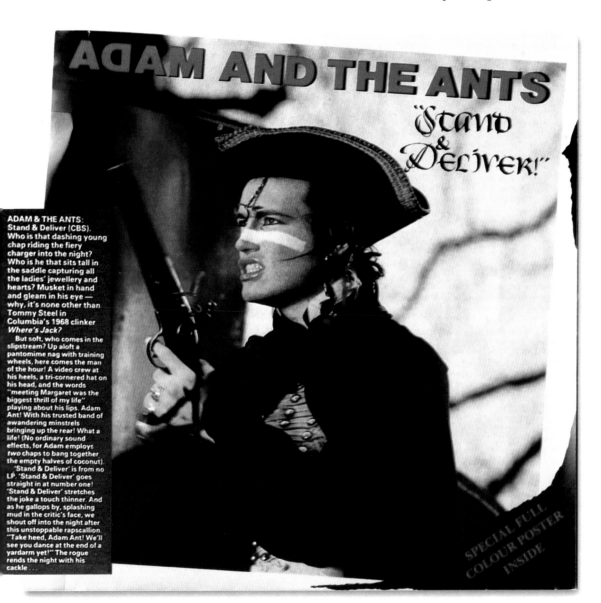

ADAM & THE ANTS: Stand & Deliver (CBS). Who is that dashing young chap riding the fiery charger into the night? Who is he that sits tall in the saddle capturing all the ladies' jewellery and hearts? Musket in hand and gleam in his eye — why, it's none other than Tommy Steel in Columbia's 1968 clinker *Where's Jack?*

But soft, who comes in the slipstream? Up aloft a pantomime nag with training wheels, here comes the man of the hour! A video crew at his heels, a tri-cornered hat on his head, and the words "meeting Margaret was the biggest thrill of my life" playing about his lips. Adam Ant! With his trusted band of awandering minstrels bringing up the rear! What a life! (No ordinary sound effects, for Adam employs *two* chaps to bang together the empty halves of coconut).

'Stand & Deliver' is from no LP. 'Stand & Deliver' goes straight in at number one! 'Stand & Deliver' stretches the joke a touch thinner. And as he gallops by, splashing mud in the critic's face, we shout off into the night after this unstoppable rapscallion. "Take heed, Adam Ant! We'll see you dance at the end of a yardarm yet!" The rogue rends the night with his cackle . . .

ADAM AND THE ANTS

"Stand & Deliver!"

SPECIAL FULL COLOUR POSTER INSIDE

84

Under The Moon Of Love
Showaddywaddy

Release Date: 6.11.76
No. Weeks In Chart: 15
Reached No. 1: 4.12.76
Total Sales: 985,000

The cartoon teddy-boy image, the famous 'walking in circles' dance routines and heart-throb status of joint vocalist Dave Bartram made the band a chart staple.

This revivalist octet formed in 1973 from the amalgamation of The Choise and covers band The Golden Hammers, who had played on the same bill many times at Leicester's Fosse Way pub. Their big break came after being runner-up in the prime-time talent show *New Faces*, which also unearthed other stars of the future such as Lenny Henry.

Showaddywaddy's initial releases were all self-penned, with 'Hey Rock 'n' Roll' reaching No. 2. They enjoyed their greatest success with catchy pop versions of US rock 'n' roll classics, such as 'Under the Moon of Love' and 'Heartbeat'. In the mid-'70s they enjoyed fifteen Top 20 hits, this particular success coming in late '76, the year in which music history tells us punk broke. Showaddywaddy still play in excess of 100 gigs a year. They could also boast a drummer with the greatest name in music – the Antiguan-born Romeo Challenger.

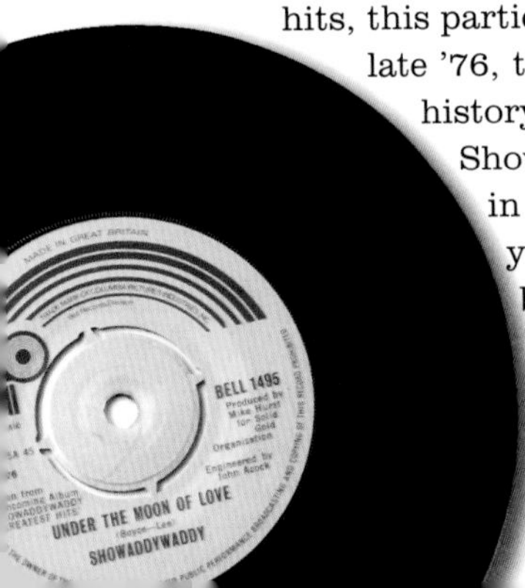

BELL 1495

UNDER THE MOON OF LOVE
SHOWADDYWADDY

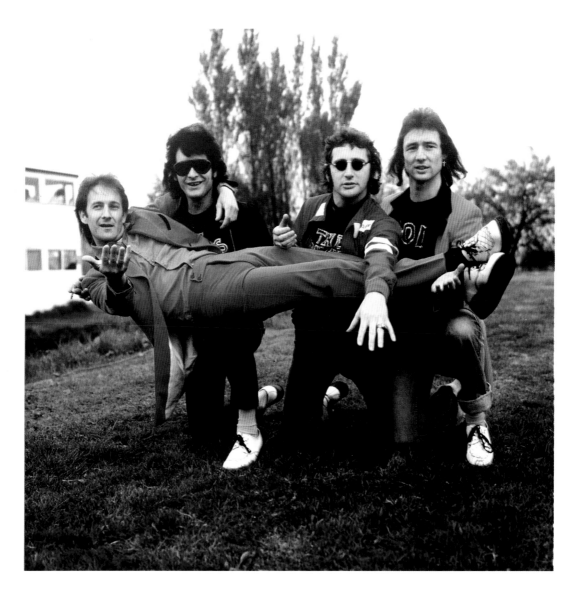

MTV

and the Birth of Video

On 1 August 1981, MTV was launched. It seems hard now to imagine that the most-watched television channel in the world did not exist before this date, such has been its pivotal role in the evolution of music and popular youth culture over the past twenty years.

At the time of its launch, its set-up cost of $30 million seemed a hefty price to pay for the lashings of soft-metal videos featuring rockers with permed hair and cavorting, scantily clad models.

Now, with its heavy rotation of hip-hop, rap, dance and alternative music, the full impact of MTV is hard to over-estimate. For, with music

television, came the birth of the whole 'promo' video industry. The new form of music video represented a complete turnaround from the traditional relationship between moving images and music.

Of course, there had been much earlier offerings. Since human beings have played musical instruments, musical scores have been

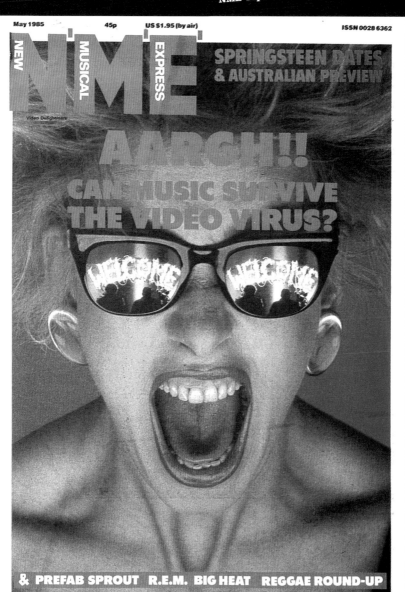

May 1985   45p   US $1.95 (by air)   ISSN 0028 6362

NEW MUSICAL EXPRESS

SPRINGSTEEN DATES
& AUSTRALIAN PREVIEW

Video Delphonare

AARGH!!
CAN MUSIC SURVIVE
THE VIDEO VIRUS?

WELCOME   WELCOME

& PREFAB SPROUT R.E.M. BIG HEAT REGGAE ROUND-UP

used to enhance the emotional impact of all manner of art forms, from ballet to theatre. From the late nineteenth century onwards, musicians were commissioned to compose pieces specifically to provide background colour to films that, until the late 1920s, would necessarily be silent. At first, there would have been a proper live band, then later a sound recording. With the birth of the 'talkies', music began fully to assume its role within the artistic character of a film.

Way back in 1921, the German composer Oskar Fischinger started to film short abstract movies to accompany musical compositions he had already written; the pieces were mainly in the classical and jazz genres (Fischinger later wrote for Disney's musical epic *Fantasia*). Similarly, from the mid-twentieth century, musicians often found themselves writing scores for screen advertisements and television shows, so a duality and natural affinity has always been there.

In the '40s, video jukeboxes were placed in public places and featured black-and-white clips of popular songs. In the '60s, similar technology led to stars such as Paul Anka (see No. 44) and Procul Harum recording their own brief video clips. At the time, artists complained of the cost of shooting these new clips – around $125 per song.

More recently, people have looked to Queen's seminal 'Bohemian Rhapsody' clip. But even before that, The Beatles had used stills from their films, and The Monkees also aired specially produced one-minute slices of music and film. Elsewhere, The Who and the Kinks

dabbled with video footage, albeit mostly rather left of field, but the trend found little interest among a public brought up on a diet of live performance. Music historian Alan Cross highlights Captain Beefheart's promotional film for his album *Lick My Decals Off, Baby* as one of the first true videos. Then, in 1975, Bruce Gower shot his aforementioned video for 'Bohemian Rhapsody' (see No. 3) and gave birth to the modern music video.

MTV was not, however, the first station to show such videos – ex-Monkee Michael Nesmith ran a cable channel doing just that called *Popclips*. On MTV's launch, there were industry predictions of the death of radio (the new station's first promo video was Buggles' 'Video Killed The Radio Star'). Time would prove them wrong, although MTV did affect the previously all-conquering influence of radio. Prior to MTV, artists placed much of their focus on their songs and live shows.

The need for a manicured, controlled visual image had always been there, but had never before been so under the microscope. With MTV, suddenly pop stars felt that they were more often reliant on how they looked than on how they sounded. Previously, radio playlists could make or break a star's career; today, while this remains the case, a poor radio airing contrasted by super-strong MTV coverage might just still work.

In some instances, music television has proved so powerful in helping to break a band that they could find themselves on top of the world charts before playing a single gig – the Spice Girls are a case in point. In America,

here there is no true national radio and there
are no weekly music papers, MTV stepped into
the role with aplomb. Inevitably, certain acts
benefited more than others did.

Early bands quick to pick up on the power of
MTV included Duran Duran, whose epic, super-
expensive videos ('Wild Boys') were mini-films
for the small screen. In the late '80s, the Stock,
Aitken and Waterman stable of former soap
stars such as Kylie and Jason were perfectly
telegenic, ready-made MTV stars (see No. 86).

Likewise, the seemingly unstoppable rise of
boy bands – Take That, Boyzone, Backstreet
Boys, N*Sync and many more – enjoys
enormous currency with the MTV audience.
Yet, paradoxically, the astronomical costs of
launching a new boy band to win MTV favour –
said to be well in excess of £1 million – has
blunted the music industry's eagerness to take
a leap of faith with a new artist, unless a sure-
fire return on the sizeable investment is more
or less guaranteed.

Michael Jackson is perhaps the most famous
producer of music videos – his mini-movie for
'Thriller' remains a classic, and its impact at
the time should not be underestimated. Since
then, he has spent exorbitant amounts on both
superb videos ('Scream') and also rather less
entertaining efforts ('Earth Song', see No. 69).
Jackson can also claim to have broken down
the racial barriers of a till-then predominantly
white MTV. Since when, its popular *Yo! MTV
Raps* slot and subsequent wholesale
championing of hip-hop, moderate gangsta rap
and garage has at least seen the spectrum of
music represented there even out.

The arrival of Nirvana's 'Teen Spirit' and the
onset of grunge changed MTV's aesthetic
overnight. Gone were the bikinis, the soft
rockers, the airbrushed videos by ageing
artists and the middle-of-the-road music. In
came Nirvana, Hole, Pearl Jam, Soundgarden
and with them the floodgates opened.
Suddenly, the alternative music world had a
voice on MTV, too. Although many critics of
MTV express their boredom with the screen
saturation by manufactured bands and
lightweight pop, the station does provide
shows such as *120 Minutes* plus countless 'MTV
Specials' on more cutting-edge artists.

One of the key aims of the music industry in
the '80s when it championed MTV was to help
stop the then fad of taping records without
actually buying them; where the music
industry will go next if the rampant MP3
burning craze does not abate is anyone's guess.

Each year, the award ceremonies that MTV
hosts are watched by tens of millions of people
worldwide; and if a band finds itself with so-
called 'heavy rotation' on MTV, it usually
follows that the charts are conquered soon
after. The brand that is MTV is perhaps now as
powerful as any the television world has seen
with its colossal franchise penetrating all
corners of the globe.

MTV has also brought us the 'unplugged'
concept, *Beavis and Butthead*, *The Real World*
and, most successfully of all, the reality soap
The Osbournes. Despite its early doubters, at
the start of the twenty-first century MTV is
recognised – rightly – as one of the most
important stations in television history.

85 Torn
Natalie Imbruglia

Release Date: 8.11.97
No. Weeks In Chart: 17
Reached No. 1: N/A
Total Sales: 982,324

The chart environment at the time was ripe for rich rewards for female artists such as Alanis Morissette and Meredith Brooks.

Known initially to millions as 'Beth' in Aussie soap institution *Neighbours*, Imbruglia had first pursued a career in tap and ballet. Her progress at a local school for performing arts was soon distracted, however, by a series of high-profile and successful Australian adverts for brands such as Coca-Cola and Bubblicious gum. She quickly tired of her subsequent two-year role in *Neighbours* and left the soap to pursue new avenues.

Decamping to London, Imbruglia spent two years in limbo, turning to songwriting and music to express her predicament. A demo of this future surprise smash single 'Torn' made its way on to RCA's desks and, with the aid of a veritable line-up of studio veterans – Phil Thornalley (ex-Cure), Nigel Godrich (Radiohead), Mark Goldenberg (Eels) and Mark Plati (David Bowie, Deee-Lite) – she recorded the accompanying hit album, *Left of the Middle*. Imbruglia enjoyed four Top 20 hits in twelve months.

Imported into America via LA radio stations, the single subsequently became one of the most aired songs in the world and it scooped a hatful

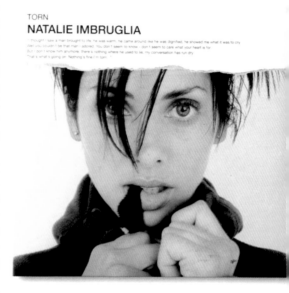

TORN
NATALIE IMBRUGLIA

of awards. 'Torn' was also a massive European hit. Several high-profile boyfriends (Lenny Kravitz, *Friends*' David Schwimmer) could not boost the rather muted sales of the follow-up album, *White Lillies Island*.

NATALIE IMBRUGLIA — talentless ex-*Neighbours* hyperbabe from the land of the bar-b-q or genuine singer/songwriter with a big bag of tunes? It's make your mind up time. For those about to Ayers Rock: SIMON WILLIAMS (words) JAMES & JAMES (photos)

N ow, this is what we in the trade would call a real Turkish Delight. For, over there, sitting demurely in the corner of a moodily-lit room, smothered in cushions and festooned with sensual trinkets from the Middle East, is a 'lady' who has been sending any normal testosterone-thrilled young 'man' quite literally stir-fry crrrrazy over the past few months.

You can't have missed the video of her worryingly addictive hit single, 'Torn', where she looks like the coy, coquettish floppy-fringed next-door neighbour of fantasy. Neither can you have avoided the incessant titbits of gossip about her peppering the tabloids as our whopping Wapping pals strive to suss out which celebrity beau is currently (harrumph!) raising her soufflé. Because she's been here. She's been there. In fact, she has been everything-and-here – even as far as London Shepherd's Bush Empire.

"I saw Bjork! She was incredible!"

Yeah?

"Yeah! But shall I tell you something funny?"

Please do!

"My friend got me a really good seat in the royal box thing and this woman in a big fur coat came and sat next to us and there was this... she about her, and I gave her this, like, look and she goes, 'Oh, excuse me!' And then I realised who it was."

"It was Madonna! And she almost sat on me! And I'd pulled a face at her!"

At this fun-sized memory, those big dizzy Disney eyes twinkle mirthfully. Are they blue? Are they green? Are they merely liquid pools of wonderment in which to dive and then drown, rather like an unearned kitten in a carrier bag? And frankly, who gives a shit? Hey, hey, hey! We're having breakfast with Natalie Imbruglia!

B REATHE IN, BREATHE OUT AND relax. For what you have just witnessed is actually a porky prime cut from the recently founded 'Oops, sorry I am just come' school of journalism. Clever, eh? Yes indeed. Thanks to the sterling work of our chums over in Glossy Mag Land, us '90s boys are now liberated sorts, entirely free to call a spade a spade and a bird a bird. Thanks to them, we've been privileged to have seen Jayne Middlemiss' navel, Zoe Ball's cleavage! Louise Nurding's spleen!! Anna Friel's bum?! And when they aren't slapping barely concealed tits on their front covers, they're putting on

Chris Evans! I thangyoo.

The age of the low-rent media yahoo is upon us. Heartily encouraged by editors obviously convinced their readership consists of semi-detta morons, the publishing world has manufactured a generation of Hyperbabes for our delectation and their sexy saucy figures. Less stuck up than her big supermodel sister, the Hyperbabe spends her days as an entertainer, her nights as a possed-up disco ducky, her treatments going 'Pheeooaaarrr!!' over some hunky slab of soccer meat and all the bits in between being fawned over by slack-jawed hacks who spend the majority of their time boasting about hanging with low-rent media yahoo Hyperbabes.

Natalie Imbruglia is supremely qualified in the Hyperbabe stakes.

Firstly, she used to be a television personality courtesy of a stint in Neighbours. Secondly, 'Torn' is enduring love affair with the Top Ten has turned her into a bona-fide pop star. And thirdly, fourthly and fifthly, she's been spotted at Blur's aftershow in Dublin (cool), been romantically linked with an MP (kooky!)

and, as we've heard, almost been used as an armchair by Ms Ciccone herself (almost neo-classical Hyperbabe behaviour). She is indeed the Oogly 'Broogly Woogly chickette from down under. Just one snagette, then: where the saucy, sizzlin' super scanteasy shelf-bustin' swimwear shots in Lad Monthly, Naz? After all, everyone keeps

telling us yer gorgeous, right?

"The record company talked to me about image and I thought, 'I'm not gonna pull it off – they're gonna see right through me!'" she sighs, toying with an exotic coffee. "So the only way I could pull it off was to be myself, otherwise they'll be able to tell that I'm bluffing.

"I went on some kids' show recently and they played 'Torn' and then they

went. 'You're wearing the same army pants as you did in the video!', and I thought, 'F—ing hell, people pay attention!' But it has worked to my advantage: people say, 'Oh, you haven't got your kit off!' But it's just easier being myself instead of having to worry about whether or not I'm 'authentic'."

It's hard to imagine Natalie Imbruglia being more 'authentic' than this. The location rather grandly described as a Turkish Delight earlier is in fact a bar off

"I SAW BJORK AND THIS WOMAN IN A BIG FUR COAT CAME AND SAT NEXT TO US. SHE ALMOST SAT ON TOP OF ME! AND I GAVE HER THIS, LIKE, *LOOK* AND SHE GOES, 'OH, EXCUSE ME!'… IT WAS MADONNA!"

Regents Street. Enticingly mystical it may be during the hours of darkness, but at 10.30 in the bloody morning ("I'm never up this early," she winces) it's a thoroughly shabby environment. To be blunt, with the pair of us on different sofas separated by a round gold table while the staff clatter about preparing for the lunchtime trade, the whole experience feels unnervingly akin to doing a TV interview in a brothel.

The reason for our sleepyheaded rendezvous is simple: Natalie is due to spend her afternoon in the even less salubrious surroundings of King's Cross, in rehearsal with her band. Which of course is extremely silly, because Natalie used to be a Soapster and, as the accompanying panel so vehemently proves, Soapsters who become singers have scant need for 'bands'. How aware were you of the history of the soap/pop interface, El Imbrooglio?

"Oh, completely aware!"

And when you left the TV show and embarked upon a musical journey didn't you think, 'Of all the career changes I could possibly do in the entire world, this would be the worst'?

"Oh, absolutely! I committed the biggest sin. It was like, OK, I've really lost my mind now!"

• Splendid. And here's where it starts to get strange. Because while Natalie has proved that it is not difficult to join the legion of singing Soapsters, her recent debut album 'Left Of The Middle' also demonstrates that it isn't particularly hard to beat 'em, either. A surprisingly cool, relevant record – suggest to El Natoo that it's less bitter than Bjork, less overwrought than Portishead and less ferocious than Garbage and she will nod and gurgle merrily – the critical and commercial response to her debut has

fun than Rag Week in the Rompy Pumpy Studey Union.

"My mum used to take me along to be an extra on film sets," she recalls, matter-of-factly. "I saw it all, how those people worked together, and there is a big difference between a film and a soap. With a film there's a beginning, a middle and an end – it's like making an album. With a soap you walk in and there are people who have been working there for 20 years, since the building

opened! It was so corporate. You had to check in and check out – it was like a normal job! It was not creative. I may as well have been doing something else."

Yeah! Like building roads, right?

"I was doing that anyway, sweetie."

Yeah! Eh?

"I was a brickie." What??! "I was supposed to be building houses on the show. I remember one time in the middle of winter I had to fall into a trench. They had a stunt guy there and I was going, 'Where's my double? What? There is no double??!' So this guy's showing me this plank of wood and this muddy, wet trench and how I fall into it. And I fall into this wet trench and then they go, 'Don't

"*NEIGHBOURS* WAS CORPORATE. YOU HA[...] IN AND CHECK OUT – A NORMAL JOB! IT W[...] CREATIVE. I MAY AS BEEN DOING SOMETH[...]"

get out! We've got to move the cameras for the next shot!' And I'm lying there thinking, 'Do I really want to do this?'"

Did you die in a horrible soapy type accident when you left and they had to kill your character off?

"No, I got married and sent off to Perth." Pause. "Same thing, really…"

H OWEVER, IN REAL LIFE, NATALIE Imbruglia's tenure in Australia was coming to an end. A solo jaunt around Kenya was followed by a move

to London, where she partied like… well, like it was 1994, actually. She schmoozed. She boozed. She oozed good time vibes. She 'lived a fantasy' in her mind. She soaked up London. Indeed, she bled it dry, to the point where "it started to shrivel". And then she got depressed.

"My career wasn't exactly peaking," she acknowledges, brusquely. "My finances were going down the toilet, and London is a tough place to live in the winter when things aren't going your

BAR-B GIRL

86 Especially For You
Kylie Minogue and Jason Donovan

Release Date: 10.12.88
No. Weeks In Chart: 14
Reached No. 1: 7.01.89
Total Sales: 982,000

Kylie and Jason were perfect for Stock, Aitken and Waterman's so-called 'Hit Factory'.

At the forefront of the Stock, Aitken and Waterman (a.k.a. PWL) chart domination of the late '80s, both Kylie and Jason capitalised on their high profile in the Australian soap *Neighbours*. As former Bananarama, Divine and Dead or Alive producers, PWL possessed an uncanny ability to release hit after hit, enjoying a track in the Top 40 continually between early 1987 and mid-1990.

Kylie's debut UK single, 'I Should Be So Lucky', was turned down by all the major labels, but proved to be the first of thirteen successive UK Top Ten singles – her debut album sold two million. This sugar-sweet ballad was PWL's fifth recording with the diminutive Minogue, teaming up with her on-screen husband (and real life boyfriend) Jason. Its release coincided with their respective characters getting married in *Neighbours* and was a sure-fire No. 1.

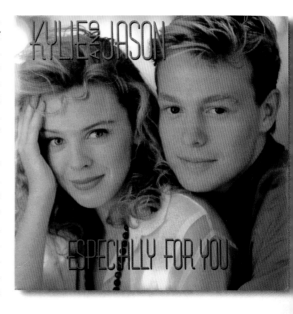

Kylie had a rather indifferent career for much of the '90s, before her re-emergence at the start of the new millennium as one of the most successful female singers in UK chart history. Jason's debut album *Ten Good Reasons* was the best-seller of 1989; but after he went to court in a notorious libel case against *The Face* (concerning his supposed sexual orientation) and plunged into cocaine addiction, his 'success' seemed at polar opposites to Minogue's. The birth of his first child saw him sober up, appear in *Joseph and his Technicolour Dreamcoat* and find much support among a British public still fond of Scott and Charleen.

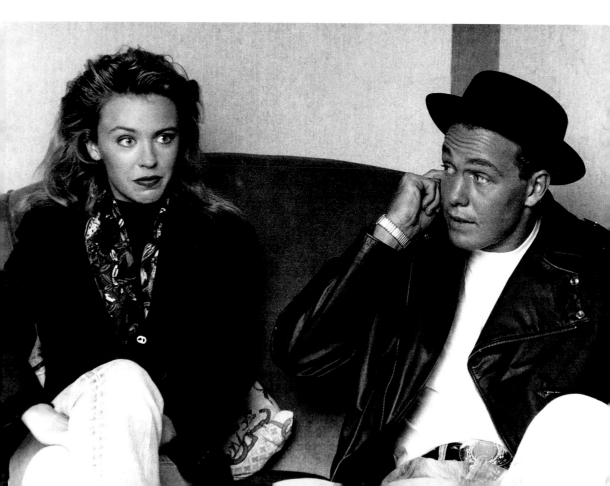

87 Hit Me With Your Rhythm Stick
Ian Dury and The Blockheads

Release Date: 9.12.78
No. Weeks In Chart: 20
Reached No. 1: 27.01.79
Total Sales: 979,100

The Blockheads provided the perfect musical accompaniment to Dury's masterful, incisive and insightful lyrics.

This funky, spliced-rock classic represented the commercial peak for an artist whose almost universal critical acclaim was, unfortunately, rarely matched by his chart successes.

A latecomer to the charts at the age of 35, Ian Dury seemed perennially oblivious to the fashions of the day (at that time, either bondage trousers or disco gear). As a result, he was seen by many as a lonely beacon of integrity. 'Hit Me With Your Rhythm Stick' provided him with his only stay at the top of the chart pile, although he was to have a handful of other chart hits.

Dury became afflicted by polio at the age of seven, but his academic and creative gifts enabled him to rise above the constraints of his disability and establish himself as a highly idiosyncratic talent. Upminster-bred, Dury studied at the Royal College of Art under Peter Blake and then taught art until his late twenties.

Inspired by his idol Gene Vincent (to whom he later penned a tribute), he then started his down-to-earth 'pub rock' band, underground favourites Kilburn and the High Roads.

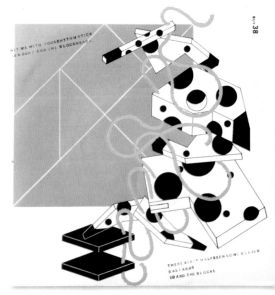

Their successor, The Blockheads, provided the perfect musical accompaniment for Dury's uniquely imaginative and insightful lyrics. Limping around on the stage, proudly sporting his polio stick, the eternal misfit Dury delivered his lyrics in his inimitable Cockney tone and

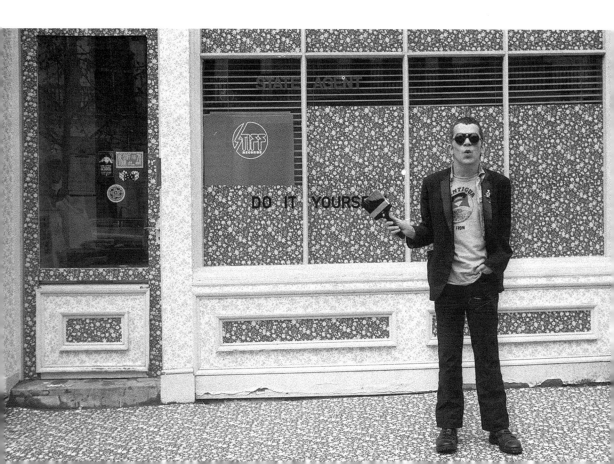

slang – 'Hit Me With Your Rhythm Stick' even contains several lines of German and French spoken/sung in a Cockney accent. This single was just one of a rash of brilliantly witty, sensitive and musically gifted songs penned by Dury and cohort Chaz Jankel. Replacing its polar opposite, Village People's 'YMCA' (see No. 33), at the top spot just a month before Sid Vicious died of an overdose, 'Rhythm Stick' stayed at No. 1 for one week only, but enjoyed two further chart visits in 1985 and 1991.

Although Dury later penned a musical, *Apples*, and acted a little too (he appears in Peter Greenaway's *The Cook, The Thief, His Wife and Her Lover*), his poetic talent is best showcased by this epochal single and on the much-lauded album, *New Boots and Panties!!*, which spent a year in the charts after its release in 1977.

His acclaimed 1998 album *Mr Love Pants*, and his dignified handling of the colorectal cancer that finally killed him in 2001, cemented Dury's remarkable legacy. He is now rightly recognised as one of the UK's most original songwriters of all time.

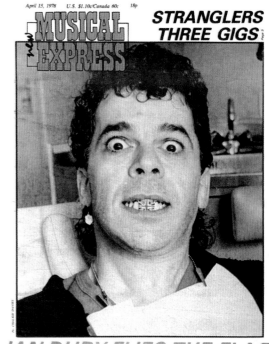

April 15, 1978   U.S. $1.10c/Canada 60c   18p

STRANGLERS THREE GIGS

IAN DURY FLIES THE FLAG

And you'd better Adam and Eve it. Billericay Dickie in the USA — Pages 31/33. Norf and Sarf job — Page 63.

'Limping around on the stage, proudly sporting his polio stick, the eternal misfit Dury delivered his lyrics in his inimitable Cockney tone and slang.'

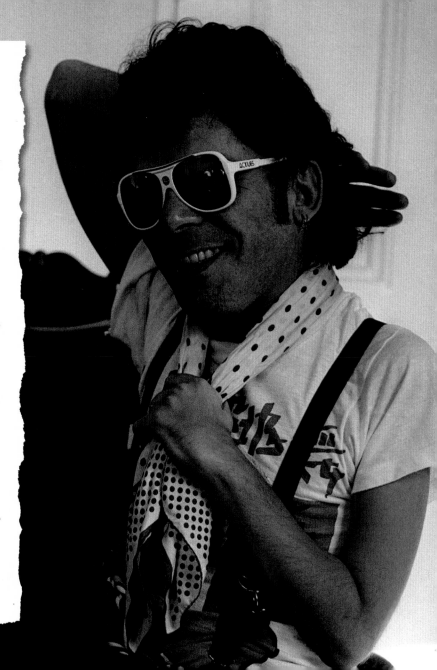

SINGLE OF THE WEEK (Act One)

IAN DURY: Hit Me With Your Rhythm Stick *(Stiff)*

A million diaries rendered redundant in the twinking of an eye! The Blockhead backlash does *not* start here. (Erasers up by ten points). So we all know of the band's chummy old pals act with the press, but no dew eyed, 'alright mate?', whacky lovable off-beat shennanegans can mask the stark truth that this record deserves no less than its full whack of the superlative stick.

It consists of geographical word wrangling over one of Chas Jankel's finest funk backings, hi hat sizzling on the beat and the Norman Watt-Roy bass bubbling like the business.

A couple of times it does seem that Dury isn't too familiar with his own lyric, but all can be forgiven because of the middle break — a bivouac awash with African jazz percussion and cranky sax runs which can tend to overshadow the rest of the single on repeated play.

The 'B' side ("There Aint Half Been Some Clever Bastards") is the offspring of "Billericay Dickie" and "England's Glory".

On Van Gogh: *"He didn't paint the Mona Lisa / That was an Italian geezer . . .".*

Empires are turned on such statements.

88

Sugar Sugar
Archies

Release Date: 11.10.69
No. Weeks In Chart: 26
Reached No. 1: 25.10.69
Total Sales: 979,000

Bubblegum pop was named after the pre-teen market it targeted, who were highlighted as the main consumer of chewing gum. And the Archies' 'Sugar Sugar' embodied it 100 per cent.

The Archies are one of the one-hit wonders of this best-selling singles list (see also No.'s 2, 60, 61, 75, 92 and 100). Masterminded by Monkees producer Don Kirschner, they were a cartoon band whose self-titled Saturday morning show on America's CBS network was a huge hit at the time.

Kirschner was rumoured to have wanted a cartoon-animated group so as to avoid the pitfalls of personality clashes that he had experienced with The Monkees.

The band represented the high point of so-called 'bubblegum' pop – a lightweight, ultra-catchy genre that spawned numerous hits in the late '60s, including this song and others such as 'Simon Says'.

The Archies' animated format is seen by many as the birth of pop-band cartoons. (Its successors included the cartoon series based on pre-teen sensations The Jackson Five and The Osmonds in the early '70s.) And all this in the year that Brian Jones died, Woodstock took place and David Bowie released his debut single, 'Space Oddity'.

The characters – Archie, Veronica, Jughead, Betty, Moose and their mascot Hot Dog – were represented on record by professional singers, the lead being taken by Ron Dante (also of The Cufflinks).

The 'group' only ever performed once, yet the six million-selling No. 1 smash 'Sugar Sugar' gave them a sufficiently high profile to open their own restaurant. Their profile in the UK was considerably lower than in the US, with only this song breaking into the charts on this side of the Atlantic.

Jonathan King later released a heavy-metal cover of the song under the moniker of Sakkarin. Dante went on to produce Barry Manilow, re-record 'Sugar, Sugar' in 1975 and become a successful Broadway producer.

'Sugar Sugar' was knocked off the top spot after eight weeks by Rolf Harris' tear-jerking 'Two Little Boys'.

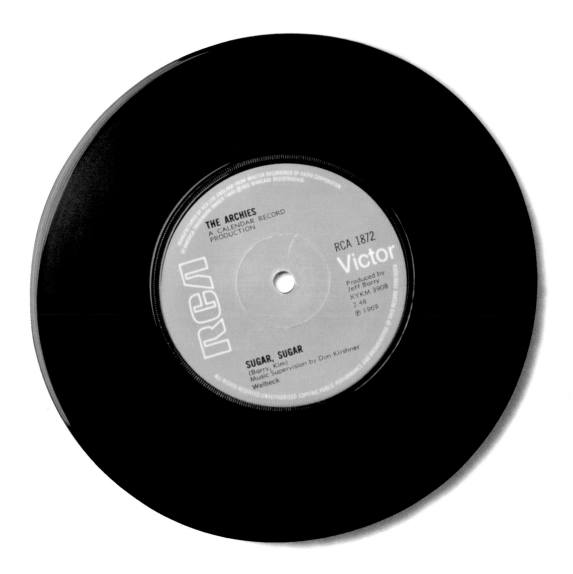

89 The Lion Sleeps Tonight
Tight Fit

Release Date: 23.01.82
No. Weeks In Chart: 15
Reached No. 1: 6.03.82
Total Sales: 978,000

Originally a South African hunting song entitled 'Mbube', early translations of the Zulu phrases mutated the key phrases into the now-familiar, albeit erroneous, 'Wimoweh' It was under that title that the trio Tight Fit made the song one of the '80s most unlikely chart-toppers.

This track was written in 1939 by Zulu singer Solomon Linda. Recorded with his group Solomon Linda's Original Evening Birds, the track sold 10,000 copies in his native country, South Africa. Legend has it that the song's lyrics were inspired by Solomon's childhood spent chasing lions away from his father's livestock.

Early on, translations of key verses in the original lyrics had twisted the Zulu words to produce the now-familiar – although linguistically incorrect – 'Wimoweh' refrain. George Weiss added full English lyrics in the early '60s.

The lycra-clad Tight Fit's 1982 hit was not the first time this deeply historical tune had been appropriated into a more popular musical medium. Both The Weavers in 1952 and folk/country-and-western quintet The Tokens in 1961 had enjoyed earlier success with their own renditions of the tune.

Indeed, The Tokens managed to notch up a million-seller in the US with their version of 'Wimoweh', re-titled 'The Lion Sleeps Tonight'. Karl Denver took the song to No. 4 in the UK the following year, while Robert John scored a Top Three US hit with it in 1972. However, Tight Fit succeeded in generating the song's loftiest UK commercial success – and also some of its worst related haircuts.

The track has proved a perennial favourite, being recorded by Ladysmith Black Mambazo, REM (as a bizarre sister track to their 'The Sidewinder Sleeps Tonite'), Jimmy Dorsey and even inspiring a 'twist' version. The tune was also the only non-Disney song performed in the Broadway production, *The Lion King*.

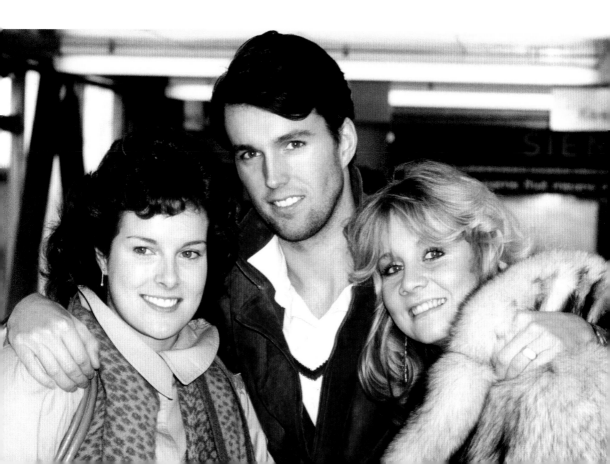

The '90s

Perhaps the most notable aspect of the '90s – a decade in which Internet and multimedia technology turned everyone's living room into a 'superhighway' of fashion, music, news and entertainment – was the global dissemination of pop culture.

During the '90s, fashion seemed to become increasingly homogeneous and, as a result, there was a real dearth of haircuts to differentiate one 'tribe' from another. Amid the rampant banality, however, there were some excellent islands for outsiders.

The leftovers of the late '80s grebo and Madchester scenes heralded the launch of the '90s, bolstered by the growing rave scene and the dayglo styles of Smiley culture. However the first great musical movement of the decade which brought with it its first youth-culture fashion, was undoubtedly grunge.

Hailing from the north-western corner of America, grunge crawled out from the Seattle underground and single-handedly changed the mechanics of the music industry. Nirvana, with their ten-million-selling *Nevermind* album

CRITISH HEAVYWEIGHT
CHAMPIONSHIP

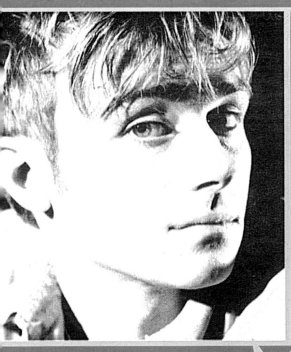

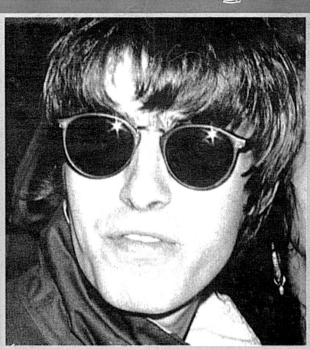

BLUR VS OASIS
UGUST 14: THE BIG CHART SHOWDOWN

were at the very core, led by their enigmatic and deeply troubled frontman Kurt Cobain. His band – pinned alongside Pearl Jam as being at the forefront of the new movement – (reluctantly) took grunge to the masses. What had started as a disparate group of bands gigging relentlessly on the underground circuit soon turned into an avalanche of multi-platinum record sales and sold-out world tours.

Older detractors derided grunge's fusion of hardcore and metal as merely re-hashing '70s rock – but this mattered little to those who were experiencing such music for the first time. There was a uniform, too – like punk before it, grunge truly was thrift-store chic. Bedecked in flannel shirts, oversized shorts cut off just below the knee and long, lanky hair, the grunge kid quickly picked up the tag of 'loser'. Girls often wore flowery dresses with thick leggings, or trousers with oversized band-logo T-shirts, rounded off with heavy boots, most often Dr Martens.

Inevitably, grunge was hijacked by the mainstream – as so many youth cultures are. Elevator music albums were released with muzak versions of grunge classics and, perhaps worst of all, fashion designers started to copy the style. The catwalks of Paris and Milan exhibited horrendous copies of the grunge look, with obscenely priced and hideously shaped versions of the thrift-store style. If this didn't kill grunge, the shot that was heard across the world – when Kurt Cobain killed himself on 8 April 1994 – did.

By then, the British music scene – previously unable to compete with the US influx – had

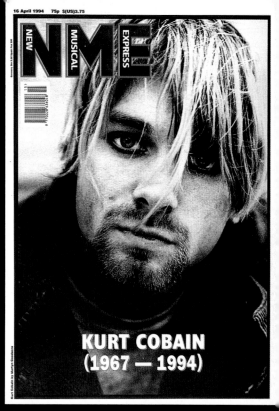

16 April 1994   75p $(US)3.75

NEW MUSICAL EXPRESS

KURT COBAIN
(1967 — 1994)

Kurt Cobain by Martyn Goodacre

already started to retaliate. The first signs had come from Suede. Set against a backdrop of slacker-driven grunge culture, Suede's songs talked of highly stylised, romantic London dramas, and frontman Brett Anderson's peculiarly camp Englishness carried the whole off to perfection.

A brief flirtation with a scene called the New Wave of New Wave reinforced the re-emergence of British talent, but it was Blur, Oasis and Pulp who signalled the full arrival of what would be christened Britpop. Blur's pivotal second album, *Modern Life Is Rubbish*, openly paraded their Anglo-centric interests. British youth put its grunge clothing away and started riffling through records by British bands once again. Cut-off shorts and plaid shirts were returned to the charity stores and long hair was cut short.

In came a variation of the casual look of the early '80s, mixed with elements of mod and other unique styles, including the occasional Hawaiian shirt. Trainers were popular, Harrington jackets made another comeback and even the Oxfam look of Pulp's Jarvis Cocker was copied by many Britpop fans.

Over the next splendid eighteen months, Pulp finally broke their fourteen-year stretch of semi-obscurity and produced a sexually subversive, comically seedy masterpiece in their first major label album *His 'n' Hers*. Elastica, Supergrass and the soon-to-be global Radiohead all also made an impact on the scene.

The mod movement enjoyed an indirect boost and mini-revival as well, with the so-called Modfather, Paul Weller, enjoying some of his biggest successes to date. Elsewhere, live music experienced a resurgence, band merchandise sales rocketed and festivals were repeatedly sold out. Record shops couldn't stock enough of Britpop acts.

Of course, Britpop couldn't last. By the time Blur and Oasis were engaging in their fêted battle for the No. 1 slot, in August 1995, there were already dissenters who bemoaned the mainstream prostitution of the scene – just like glam, punk, grunge and many others before it. By mid-1996, with most of the major Britpop

players recording new material or on sabbaticals, the movement was effectively dead.

But the '90s, post-Britpop, still had much to offer. Gangsta rap and hip-hop enjoyed their most fruitful commercial years, turning artists such as Puff Daddy into multi-millionaire tycoons and late rappers like Tupac Shakur and B.I.G. into icons. The tail end of the decade saw Eminem become the biggest-selling solo artist in the world, with a trio of exceptional albums forged around his highly controversial Slim Shady alter ego.

Naturally, rap and hip-hop fashion seeped into the mainstream, becoming so prevalent as to give birth to the parody of comedian Ali G. Rap's early offerings in the late '70s had included the seminal 'Rapper's Delight' by The Sugarhill Gang and 'The Message' by Grandmaster Flash.

Now rap offered up the skills of LL Cool J, Public Enemy, NWA, Run-D.M.C., Beastie Boys, Ice-T, Ice Cube and a host of other brilliant wordsmiths, to make it the most innovative and enthralling genre of the decade. The excesses of gangsta rap and the over-commercialisation of hip-hop in the latter half of the '90s should not detract from the essential importance of the development.

Maybe the '90s *were* notable for the fact that there were no silly haircuts any more – but closer inspection reveals a proliferation of exciting fashions and musical developments. Even the last days of the decade brought yet more change, with the street-to-screen success of So Solid Crew – bringing with it a torrent of superb UK garage.

90 The Next Time/Bachelor Boy
Cliff Richard and The Shadows

Release Date: 6.12.62
No. Weeks In Chart: 18
Reached No. 1: 3.01.63
Total Sales: 976,000

Sir Cliff once held the record for being both the youngest and the oldest performer to earn a No. 1 success, with 'Living Doll' (1959) and 'The Millennium Prayer' (1999) respectively.

This track was Cliff's first co-writing credit and only his second single in this book, after the million-selling 'The Young Ones' (see No. 68). Again taken from a musical movie, _Summer Holiday_, both tracks from this double A-side single were first performed at the then hugely popular show _Sunday Night at the Palladium_.

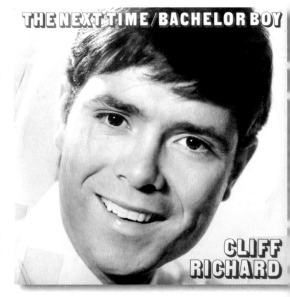

Premiering at the top of the charts, 'The Next Time/Bachelor Boy' was surrounded by associated acts: it was displaced after three weeks by The Shadows' 'Dance On', which in turn was replaced by the debut duet of ex-Shadows Jet Harris and Tony Meehan, 'Diamonds'. Five weeks later, Cliff was back at the top with 'Summer Holiday'. The movie soundtrack _Summer Holiday_ was the No. 1 album for over three months. By now, former factory clerk Cliff was an established superstar; by mid-1963, the Liverpool beat groups had arrived and to some extent taken over the charts, but Cliff's popularity remained virtually intact.

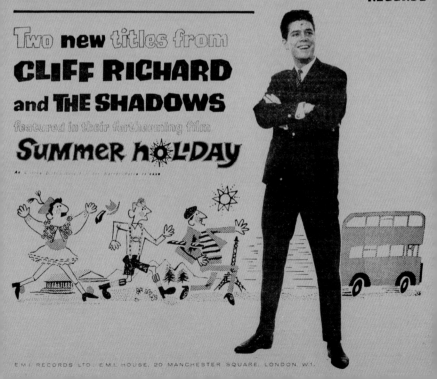

91 Fame
Irene Cara

Release Date: 3.07.82

No. Weeks In Chart: 16

Reached No. 1: 17.07.82

Total Sales: 975,000

Cara's feel-good electrifying alto voice and energised instrumentation on this single sold it by the truckload.

The inspiration for a million matching sets of leg-warmers and leotards, Irene Cara's role in the Alan Parker box-office smash movie *Fame* came after a childhood spent on Broadway (*Maggie Flynn*), in national television series (*Electric Company* and *Roots: The Next Generation*) and in movies (*Sisters*). By the age of ten, she had performed on stage with Stevie Wonder, Sammy Davis Jr and Roberta Flack.

Her profile moved up several notches when she played Coco Hernandez, the multi-talented South Bronx youngster attending the New York High School of Performing Art in *Fame*. The movie was a huge blockbuster, set fashion trends for much of the year and proved a cultural phenomenon.

The single did not reach the UK No. 1 slot until two years after the film's release, its delayed success being due to the immense popularity of the spin-off television series. Critical applause also flooded in, with this song winning Cara an Oscar and widespread international acclaim.

Two subsequent Grammies and a second Academy Award for 'What A Feeling', from the

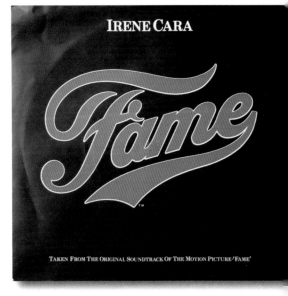

TAKEN FROM THE ORIGINAL SOUNDTRACK OF THE MOTION PICTURE 'FAME'

dance-hit film *Flashdance*, sealed a remarkably productive three years in the charts for Cara.

Since which time, Irene Cara has toured extensively, written the screen play for *A Waltz with Destiny*, formed an all-girl group called Caramel and also enjoyed a European hit with Switzerland's DJ Bobo.

FAME IS THE SPUR

Kids play UK gigs

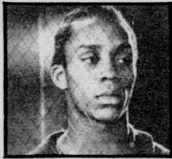

HI, LEROY!

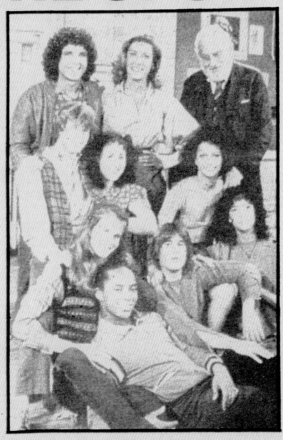

THE KIDS FROM FAME arrive in the UK right after Christmas to make their world debut concert appearances in this country. Their arrival follows hot on the heels of the enormous success of the TV series *Fame,* and the two chart-topping albums of its soundtrack. The troupe features Debbie Allen (Lydia), Lee Curreri (Bruno), Erica Gimpel (Coco), Carlo Imperato (Danny), Lori Singer (Julie) and Gene Anthony Ray (Leroy), plus ten dancers — all produced, staged and directed by Debbie Allen.

They play Brighton The Centre on December 28 (two shows at 4 and 8pm), London Royal Albert Hall on December 30 and 31 (two shows each day at 3 and 7.30pm) and Birmingham National Exhibition Centre on January 1 (one show at 7.30pm). Tickets are priced £10, £9, £7.50, £7, £5 and £3.50 (London) and £8.50, £7.50 and £6.50 (Brighton and Birmingham). Booking arrangements are as follows:

BRIGHTON: By personal application to the box-office, or by post from The Fame Box Office, P.O. Box 141, London SW6 5AS — make cheques and POs payable to "Andrew Miller Concerts Ltd." and enclose SAE. WEMBLEY: By personal application to all Keith Prowse branches, or by post from the same address as for Brighton. BIRMINGHAM: By post from The Fame Box Office, P.O. Box 4, Altrincham, Cheshire WA14 2JQ — Postal Orders only made payable to "Kennedy Street Enterprises Ltd." and enclose SAE. Or by personal application to the NEC box-office, Cyclops Sound (Birmingham), Piccadilly Records (Manchester), Mike Lloyd Records (Newcastle-under-Lyme), Goulds (Wolverhampton) or Coventry Apollo.

92 Ghostbusters
Ray Parker Jr

Release Date: 25.08.84
No. Weeks In Chart: 31
Reached No. 1: N/A
Total Sales: 974,001

The song was a last-minute addition to the film of the same name, and was only included in its present form after Aykroyd insisted on the tune being 'danceable' – initially, it had been intended as a backing track only.

This was the eponymous hit song from the then biggest-grossing comedy film ever. *Ghostbusters* **starred Bill Murray, Dan Aykroyd and Harold Ramis as a trio of chaotic ghost exterminators in New York.**

Ray Parker Jr's theme song was not his first or even his biggest-selling hit (it only ever reached No. 2 in the UK charts). Parker Jr was a veteran musician and songwriter/producer, having toured with, and played on records by, Stevie Wonder. He had also backed Gladys Knight and the Pips, as well as the Temptations – not to mention having co-written songs for Barry White and penning Rufus and Chaka Khan's US smash 'You Got the Love'. Parker's own act, Raydio, enjoyed its own US million-seller with 'Jack and Jill, You Can't Change That'.

Legal problems emerged subsequently with a lawsuit from Huey Lewis and the News. *Ghostbusters: The Musical* had a lesser impact. Parker Jr later wrote songs for, among others, New Edition, Randy Hall and Diana Ross.

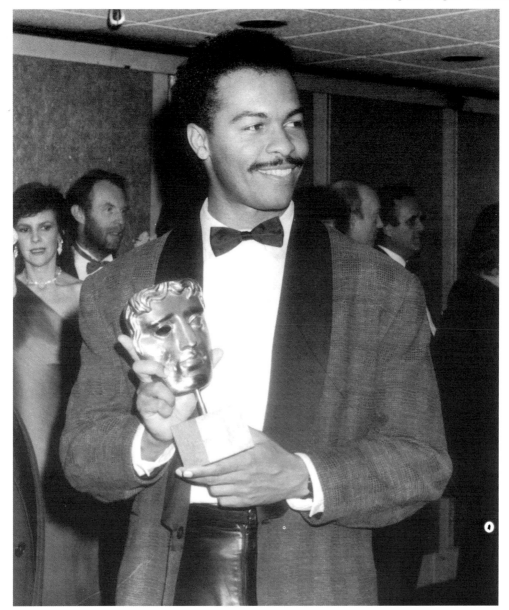

93 Uptown Girl
Billy Joel

Release Date: 15.10.83
No. Weeks In Chart: 17
Reached No. 1: 5.11.83
Total Sales: 974,000

Such was the impact of Billy Joel's smash single, 'Uptown Girl' – and the corresponding album *Innocent Man* – in raising his profile on this side of the Atlantic, that the following year he boasted no fewer than five albums in the UK charts.

This was Joel's biggest UK hit, enjoying five weeks at No. 1 and featuring his model and future second wife Christine Brinkley in the video, which was set in a mechanic's garage. 'Uptown Girl' was pulled from the smash album *Innocent Man*, which was Joel's pastiche tribute to the influences on his career. This single, heavily styled in the Four Seasons mood, was the first of several hit singles from that hit album.

Long Islander Joel was a prodigious classical pianist who had started to play at the age of four – more curiously, spurning a promising career as a boxer in order to pursue his passion for music. Various failed groups and spells as a lounge pianist and commercial jingles writer eventually led him towards a solo career in the '70s.

It was at this time that Joel first struck commercial gold, with the nine million-selling album entitled *The Stranger*. His double album, *Greatest Hits, Volumes 1 and 2 (1973–1985)*, has shifted twenty million copies in the US alone.

Although seen by many as something of an MOR artist, Joel has in fact penned numerous seminal songs, including 'Piano Man' and 'The Entertainer'. Just The Way You Are' is listed in the Rock and Roll Hall Of Fame's '500 Songs That Shaped Rock And Roll'.

Disenchantment with the pop scene and a much-publicised spell in Silver Hill Hospital in 2002 should not dim the achievements of Grammy-winning Joel's 30-year music career. In early 2001, Westlife enjoyed their own No. 1 with a charity cover of this track, which featured Claudia Schiffer in the video.

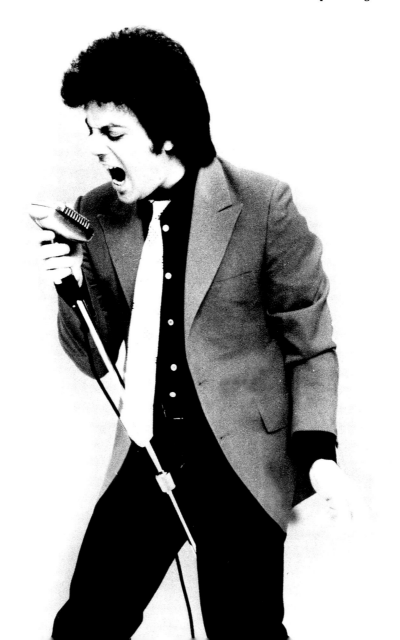

94 Ride On Time
Black Box

Release Date:	12.08.89
No. Weeks In Chart:	22
Reached No. 1:	9.09.89
Total Sales:	973,850

The Italian house cut was a huge UK smash, staying atop the charts for six weeks, only to be plagued by controversy over the sampling.

Spearheading a surge of Italian house music (or 'Italo-house') infecting the UK charts in the late '80s, Black Box was the creative *nom de plume* of three expert studio musicians: club DJ Daniele Davoli, programmer Mirko Limoni and classical musician Valeric Semplici. Using numerous pseudonyms, they had already helmed many Italian hits via their north Italian Groove Groove Melody production outfit, including work with hit Italian pop act Spagna.

The title of 'Ride On Time' came about as a result of a mishearing of the original sample – the lyric is actually 'Right on time . . . ' It was their debut release as Black Box, fronted by the striking black French model and vocalist, Katrine, whom a mutual friend had spotted at a nightclub. The single was a huge UK smash, staying on top of the charts for six weeks, only to be plagued by controversy concerning the sampling of Loleatta Holloway's late '70s disco single 'Love Sensation' (which *Billboard* magazine called, 'perhaps the most dissected, resurrected, reconstructed and restyled track of the disco era.'). Relative success in the dance wary US followed, as did a string of UK hits. A 1996 comeback album was met with a decidedl muted response.

A cover version by the Welsh act Lemo Meringue Gang, entitled 'Ride On Tea Time did not add to the near million-selling success Undeterred, however, the trio went on t produce and write for the much-maligne Vanilla Ice on his 1991 *Cool As Ice* album.

> **BLACK BOX: Ride On Time** (*RCA*)
> "It's sorta Italian House and nobody knows whether the singer is a man or a woman!" breathes RCA press officer Dave Harper. What an amusing gimmick. A high spirited and almost soulful dance track that pisses all over Belgium. Whether it pisses on Belgium from a sitting down or a standing up position is the only point to be debated.

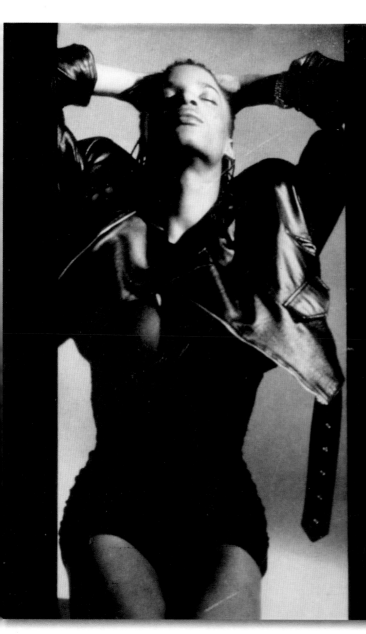

black box
ride on time

deconstruzione italiano

95 Telstar
Tornados

Release Date: 30.08.62

No. Weeks In Chart: 25

Reached No. 1: 4.10.62

Total Sales: 967,000

The brainchild of maverick independent producer Joe Meek, The Tornados' instrumental summer smash was the first song by a UK artist to hit the top spot in the US.

Inspired by televised pictures of the world's first communications satellite, the Telstar, maverick UK record producer Joe Meek created this instrumental summer smash with The Tornados. It became the first song by a UK artist to hit the top spot in the US (global sales topped five million).

The track enjoyed five weeks as the UK's No. 1 followed by six months in the charts. The enigmatic Meek was said to be tone deaf and therefore had to rely on musical cohorts, such as a young Ritchie Blackmore, to put his thoughts into sound.

The Tornados were recruited originally as Billy Fury's backing band, and included Clem Cattini, who can (uniquely) claim to have drummed on over a hundred UK chart hits.

The lead keyboard line on 'Telstar' was played on a primitive electric valve-driven organ, capable of playing only one note at a time, and the entire song was recorded on a twin-track machine.

During the period the track was being recorded, Meek also predicted – to much ridicule – that there would soon be record players which would not require a stylus . . .

The Tornados were the only instrumental group to rival the omnipresent The Shadows; however, the arrival of the vocal-driven Merseybeat rang the death knell for such acts (nonetheless, the group later recorded the *Stingray* theme tune).

A later plagiarism lawsuit troubled Meek deeply, and stalled the financial rewards of this song – five years after this hit, Meek shot his landlady and then killed himself; the date of his suicide was the eighth anniversary of Buddy Holly's death (whom Meek claimed to have contacted in seances). The Tornados still tour regularly and with great success.

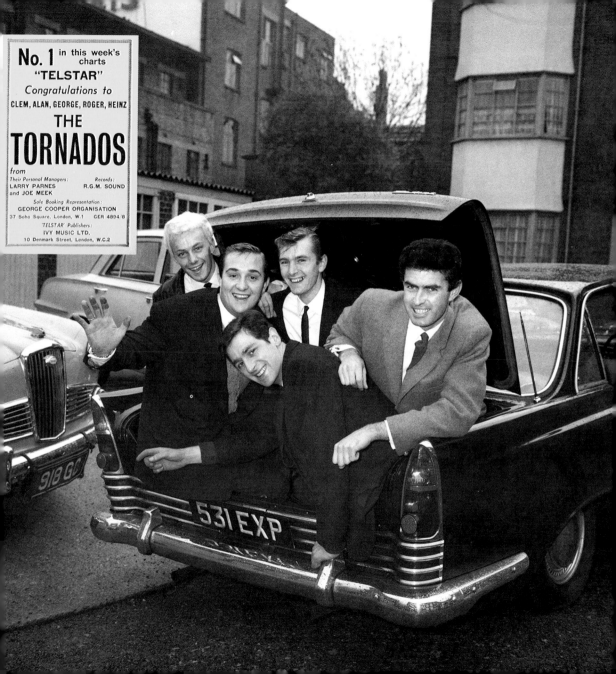

The music charts represent a cultural melting pot that is notorious for its cruel and fickle loyalties, mocking of anything that smacks of longevity and ever hungry for something new. Yet one DJ has somehow managed to outlast every fad, craze and movement – and has even helped start a few, too. That man is John Peel.

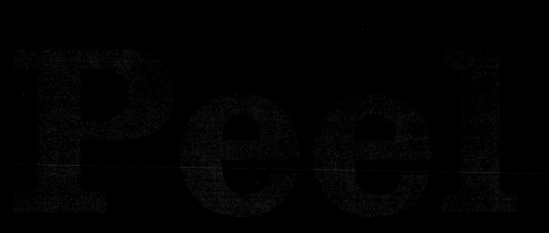

Peel's tale goes back to the very birth of rock and roll. The rock 'n' roll legend Gene Vincent was perhaps the archetypal rock rebel. In the mid-'50s, his wild antics and leather-clad persona made him a quintessential part of this fiery new medium. A motorcycle accident had left him with a permanent limp, and this disability was further exacerbated in the car crash that also took the life of Eddie Cochran. Vincent struggled thereafter, and – following a sliding career and drink problems – he died of an ulcer, aged just 36.

To a teenage John Ravenscroft, a.k.a. John Peel, Gene Vincent was incredible. Born in Heswall, near Chester, John grew up on the opposite side of the River Mersey to Liverpool, and is therefore not a Scouser at all. Yet it was this Mersey connection which would play a vital role in his future career. As a child, he would spend most of his days around the Liverpool office of his cotton-broker father, Robert 'Bob' Ravenscroft. It was nearly a decade before The Beatles. At the Liverpool Empire, John saw many of the pre-rock 'n' rollers – Johnnie Ray and Frankie Laine, and then first-generation rockers such as Duane Eddy, Eddie Cochran and Gene Vincent. After attending boarding school from the age of seven to seventeen, followed by two years of military service, John went to live in Dallas, Texas. He left for the US in 1960 – just when, ironically, Liverpool was about to take over the music world.

Because of his accent and supposed connection with The Beatles (whom he did not know), Peel got work on a Dallas Radio WWR. With his dry humour and eclectic choice of (often European) records, he quickly established a following. He was present in the immediate aftermath of the John F Kennedy assassination, telling the police that he was a reporter for *The Liverpool Echo*, and also later, just after the accused assassin, Lee Harvey Oswald, was killed in the basement of Dallas police HQ. His US radio jobs honed his DJ skills such that, on his return to the UK in 1967, he was a prime candidate for the UK pirate radio scene.

Opting for Radio London rather than the more famous Radio Caroline, Peel won critical acclaim for his unorthodox show, *The Perfumed Garden*. He has admitted that his midnight slot allowed him to tamper with the strict programme structures, abandoning adverts, news and weather to leave ample room for his choice of music.

In September 1967, the BBC launched Radio One. John Peel was superbly placed to become one of their first DJs. His initial contract was for a trial period of six weeks – he has been there ever since. His first notable show was called *Top Gear*, continuing a tradition of oddly titled programmes. Once at Radio One, Peel had access to the biggest recording stars of the day; he has since recorded almost every band of note for his legendary Peel Sessions. Almost The Beatles, The Rolling Stones and Oasis are perhaps the most high-profile absentees.

Over the past decades, Peel has been solely responsible for the first radio airing of literally hundreds of bands, yet as a 60-year-old in the new millennium, his credibility and choice of artist seems undimmed. Every week he receives in excess of 200 CDs, 60 twelve-inch singles and 20 seven-inch singles.

His favourite sessions include the punk band the Slits and a reggae outfit called Culture. Surprisingly, he recalls how the Clash complained about the standard of studio gear and informed him that they could not therefore finish the session. While music has been mutating into all its variant forms, Peel has often been the first DJ to give exposure to the new movements – he can happily claim to have lent his early support to punk, reggae, hip-hop, thousands of indie bands and many more.

Peel now commands a unique position in British rock history. At a star-studded event filled with young rock stars, often all eyes will fall on Peel, an Archers fan who lives deep in the countryside and has affectionately nicknamed his wife The Pig. He can claim to have straddled the entire lifespan of rock and roll during his radio career and will probably never be replaced at Radio One – year after year, statistics show that his show has the largest percentage of the station's young listeners. A latter-day excursion to BBC Radio Four for his show *Home Truths*

9 September 1989   55p

BIG AUDIO DYNAMITE
A night on the tiles with Mick Jones

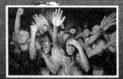

68 PAGES

NEW MUSICAL EXPRESS
NME

READING Fire and rain: mega report

Sugaring the Peel

BOBBY BROWN
Will the Jack of Swing be the next King of Soul?

BARRY WHITE
battles Steven Wells

Plus!
BLUE NILE
CHRISTY MOORE
PHRANC
ROBERT SMITH's solo LP

FESTIVE 50
John Peel's birthday bash
(starring Ian McCulloch, David Gedge, Guy Chadwick and a cast of thousands)

John Peel with (left) David Gedge of The Wedding Present, Guy Chadwick of The House Of Love and (behind) Ian McCulloch.

Picture by Bleddyn Butcher

hugely popular and diluted his rock
ot one iota.

Peel won the Sony Award for
of the Year; in 1994, he was named
ius by the *NME*. In recognition of
tion to youth culture and music he
n swamped with honorary degrees:
iversity of East Anglia (MA), the
University of East Anglia and
llam University (doctorates), John
versity Liverpool (Fellowship), not
the universities of Portsmouth and
d the Open University.

one of the most influential figures in
ic industry, Peel's own songwriting
limited to the first verse of a
Song For Europe called 'Ding Dong'
penned back in 1971. In his own
eels that 'the best songs are those
the capacity to surprise, even after
have made them apparently familiar.
things in many records which I
he very best songs are those which
acular effects or any misguided
in favour of a simple truth.'

ed about his view of songs and
, John Peel told this writer, 'If you'll
some heavy-duty name dropping, I
ndon hospital ward with John and
time of the release of *Abbey Road*.
nt a footservant out for the week's
s and I asked him why, given the
cclaim and vast sales that followed
' release, did he bother with the
eed to find out what my songs are
plied.'

🛋 ON THE COUCH

JOHN PEEL

What song describes you best? "I always think lines in
Fall songs are about me, the way that girls at Boyzone
gigs think they're looking at them… But in my melancholy
moods it would be a great Don Gibson song recorded by
Roy Orbison called 'I'd Be A Legend In My Time'."

What is heaven? "Pretty much what I'm doing now!"

What is hell? "Meetings."

What is your earliest memory? "Standing in my
bedroom, only just big enough to see out the window,
watching the sky light up from where Birkenhead and
Liverpool were burning after Nazi bombing raids."

What is your greatest fear? "Serious illness
affecting my family."

Who is your all-time hero? "Bill Shankly. He was a
great football manager and a good socialist."

What's the most trouble you've been in? "I spent
ten hours in the drunk tank in Dallas County Jail. I wasn't
drunk but I'd committed five traffic violations in the
course of a couple of miles. They used to slam you in
the drunk tank to teach you a lesson and it certainly did.
I was the only person in there who was sober; all the
other people were very violent. There was a sink, a urinal
and a toilet just stuck on the wall. If you wanted a crap
you had to have it with everybody watching you."

Who was the first love of your life? "Helen Maddox,
when I was about five."

What's your greatest talent? "I can make a noise like
a dolphin. And I'm really good at parallel parking. I keep
hoping I can find some way to combine these two
talents for commercial gain."

**Upon whom would you most like to exact revenge,
how and why?** "People who gave me a terrible time at
school. One of those people is a vicar and I have this
fantasy of turning up in his church and denouncing him.
But I think the contemplation of revenge is often more
agreeable than the actual exacting."

What's your most treasured possession? "When we
got married, Sheila had these really nicely bound books
made, with little drawings and things in. So, them."

What have you most regretted doing while drunk?
"I once found myself shagging a go-go girl in a men's
toilet, thinking, 'This is a pretty joyless business'."

What can you cook? "I can boil eggs and make toast.
I'm not proud of this at all."

What's the best piece of advice you've received?
"I don't really take advice! But my philosophy would be,
do as you would be done by."

Can you read music? "No!"

If you were invisible for a day, what would you do?
"I'd go and have a look around our village and see how
people behave when there's no-one there."

What are your final three wishes? "Long and
contented lives for my children, world peace, and
that my dad had lived longer."

Kitty Empire

PEEL GETS OBE

Veteran DJ JOHN PEEL was honoured for his services to radio broadcasting and popular music with an OBE at Buckingham Palace last week (November 26).

Peel, who was presented with the medal by Prince Charles on behalf of the Queen, said afterwards: "My dad always thought I was a bit of a dickhead. I guess he'd be really proud, so it's for him really and my mum and Sheila's *(his wife's)* mum and dad."

Andy Parfitt, controller of Radio 1, congratulated Peel and pledged to keep him on the airwaves. He said: "The John Peel phenomenon has touched all those that care about music across the generations. He's an extraordinary man, passionate, humble and very funny. My predecessor *(Matthew Bannister)* said, 'As long as there's a breath in my body, John Peel will be on Radio 1'. The same applies with me."

The investiture means Peel is now an

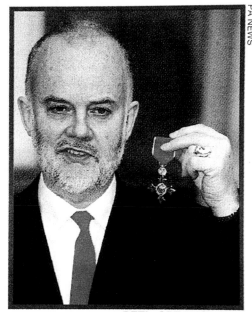

PEEL: OBE HERE NOW

Officer Of The Most Excellent Order Of The British Empire and he can put the letters OBE after his name, but it does not confer him with any other special privileges.

96 Wonderwall
Oasis

Release Date: 11.11.95
No. Weeks In Chart: 34
Reached No. 1: N/A
Total Sales: 966,940

One of the finest moments in the Gallagher brothers' back catalogue and their great break-through single.

'Wonderwall' marked a certain plateau of achievement in Noel Gallagher's maturing songwriting ability. There seemed little point in sifting through the largely meaningless lyrics, but it didn't matter: this was a truly classic song with its bluesy intonations and irresistible hooks, shamelessly filled with clusters of Beatles references – for example, it was also the title of George Harrison's first solo album, a largely experimental electronic record. For his part, Noel claimed that if you dug deeply enough, the Nirvana classic 'Smells Like Teen Spirit' lurked somewhere in the undertone of this track.

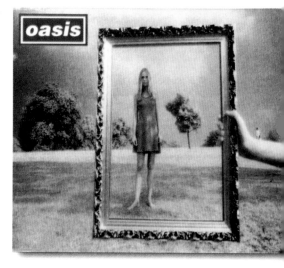

Coming at the absolute peak of Britpop, and having lost the August 1995 scuffle with Blur for the No. 1 slot, this was Oasis losing the battle but winning the war. As Britpop found its way onto the BBC News, a wash of superb British bands, such as Pulp, Elastica and Supergrass and the soon-to-be global Radiohead, plus The Bluetones and Dodgy, became household names.

However, it was Oasis and songs like 'Wonderwall' that took the fight to the US, the home of slacker culture and grunge, which had dominated the British alternative scene since 1991. Back at home, they found able assistance – not that any was needed – from a cavalry in the shape of the peculiar Mike Flowers Pops cover version of 'Wonderwall', which almost forced its easy-listening way to the top slot in Christmas of 1995. The accompanying album (What's The Story) Morning Glory? remains unsurpassed in recent British rock history.

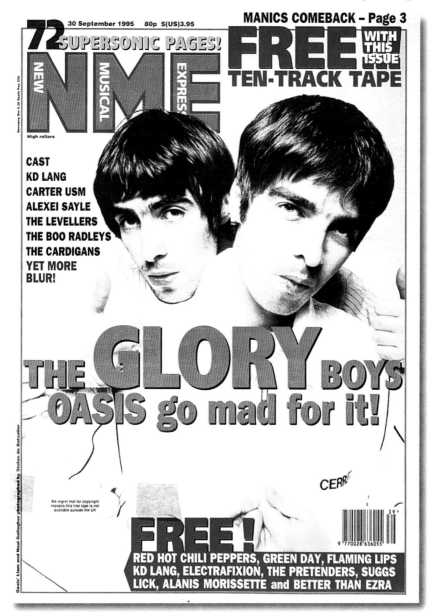

97 Amazing Grace
Royal Scots Dragoon Guards

Release Date: 1.04.72
No. Weeks In Chart: 27
Reached No. 1: 15.04.72
Total Sales: 962,000

The Royal Scots Dragoon Guards was renowned as one of the British Army's finest bands; the bandsmen initially played kettle drums and trumpets while mounted on striking grey steeds.

While music archivists argue over who was the first rock 'n' roll artist, the Royal Scots Dragoon Guards can boast a history that traces back to 1678 – quite a while before even the *NME* had thought of producing charts . . . In fact, some historians have gone so far as to attribute the birth of modern military drumming to the Royal Scots Dragoon Guards.

In combat, the regiment has distinguished itself throughout its history, seeing action at Waterloo, the Crimea, both World Wars and also during the Gulf War. When they are not on musical duty, the modern-day soldiers serve as tank crewmen.

The birth of this instrumental, bagpipe-filled hit single came about almost by chance. A version of 'Farewell to the Greys' was being recorded, the release of which was planned to coincide with the amalgamation of several different regiments. As an after-thought, Bandmaster Fairburn and Pipe Major Pryde suggested that the regiment play 'Amazing Grace', a traditional eighteenth-century hymn.

After the recording was complete, legend has it that all present knew immediately that something very special had been captured. When a late night BBC Radio Two programme casually aired the tune some time later, its phone lines became jammed with calls from delighted listeners, and a phenomenon had begun.

Remarkably, the song – which also provided a hit in the early '70s for singer-songwriter Judy Collins – topped the charts for five weeks in 1972 and led to the release of a rash of 'copycat' military records. Sadly, the band – which, as 'The Pipes and Drums and Military Band of the Royal Scots Dragoon Guards', could boast one of the longest titles of any recording artist – was absorbed into another, larger unit in 1994.

DRAGOON GUARDS FOR FREE HYDE PARK GIG

THE FIRST FREE open-air concert of the year in London's Hyde Park will be held on Sunday, May 7 — but it won't be a rock event. The concert features the Royal Scots Dragoon Guards Band, who will be giving their first public performance in this country since "Amazing Grace" entered the chart. The band is currently stationed in Germany and is flying to London specially for the concert. Meanwhile, it was learned this week that their No. 1 hit has already sold nearly 400,000 copies within four weeks of release.

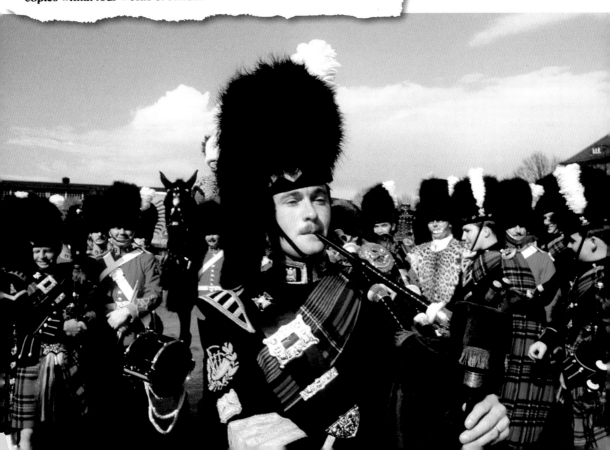

98

Back For Good
Take That

Release Date: 8.04.95
No. Weeks In Chart: 13
Reached No. 1: 8.04.95
Total Sales: 959,582

Initially, their homoerotic-styled imagery and Hi-NRG dance music appealed to the gay scene but, gradually, the female teen market turned Take That into all-powerful chart toppers.

Coming after the domination of slacker-led grunge and just before the chirpy irony of Britpop were Take That: five Manchester-based young men whose model good looks and accomplished songwriting (courtesy of Gary Barlow) turned them into Europe's biggest band in the early to mid-'90s.

They released seven singles before their first No. 1, 'Pray', in 1993; 'Back For Good' was their sixth out of a total of eight chart toppers. Taking their name from a headline about Madonna, the band and their mentor Nigel Martin-Smith aimed to be the UK's answer to America's commercially mammoth New Kids On The Block.

This subtle yet infectious ballad, perhaps Barlow's classiest composition and winner of many songwriting awards, was possibly their artistic swansong, selling 300,000 in its first week. Although future singles also hit No.1, the departure of former double-glazing salesman Robbie Williams – who spiralled into drugs and alcohol before emerging phoenix-like to become

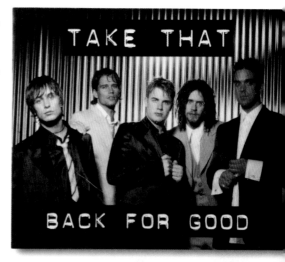

Britain's premier male solo star – and the rise of Britpop, spearheaded by Blur and Oasis, sealed the band's fate. On their demise in 1996, charity phonelines reported record numbers of distraught young fans calling to seek solace.

TAKE THAT
Back For Good *(RCA)*

PROPER SONG alert! I dunno about you, but what I want from Take That is rippling pants, jumping around and Lulu at the end. 'Back For Good' is just too classy, too like a Cliff Richard Christmas adult ballad about how he misses the wife he's never actually had, and what a painful thing divorce, which he's never actually had, is. As for The Beatles medley recorded Live!, tacked on the end – don't they know The Beatles were shite? Everyone knows that.

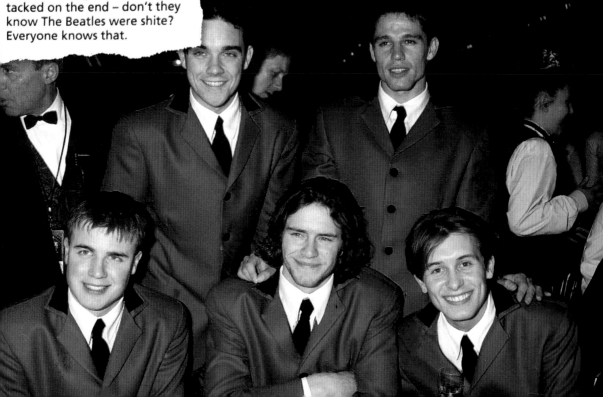

99 Sailing
Rod Stewart

Release Date: 16.08.75

No. Weeks In Chart: 34

Reached No. 1: 6.09.75

Total Sales: 955,000

This single effectively signalled the death knell of The Faces, who split up the month after its release. Still, it racked up sales of nearly one million – not bad for the son of a north London newsagent.

A model-railway enthusiast and one-time professional football apprentice, Rod Stewart is one of the world's most successful artists. 'Sailing' was Rod's first No. 1 in three years, and came amid a commercial purple patch that coincided with a hectic period in his private life.

Originally, the Gavin Sutherland-penned song was a No. 1 for four weeks, starting in mid-September 1975, only to re-enter at No. 3 after being used as the theme tune for the TV show *Sailor*, set on board the aircraft carrier *HMS Ark Royal*. The corresponding *Atlantic Crossing* album was also a chart topper for the singer formerly known as Rod The Mod.

Previously, Rod had been juggling his solo career with his role in The Faces, resulting in a remarkable run of eight critically lauded albums in the space of only four years (seen by many as Rod's best work). In the mid-'70s he enjoyed six consecutive million-selling albums.

By late 1975, artists such as Rod were detested by the new punk generation, but his commercial power remained seemingly unaffected by the snarling sea change that was taking place in the music scene.

When his hit single 'Sailing' was released, Rod was in the midst of a high-profile affair with actress Britt Ekland (one of a string of blonde paramours). He was also rumoured to be having problems with the Inland Revenue and to be on the point of relocating to Los Angeles (although a proud Scot, Rod was actually born in London).

Surprisingly – for a famed rock strutter who later wore leopard skin, chest-revealing leotards and make-up – Rod's stage fright was once quite debilitating. At one show, it became so severe that this future world-class performer had to sing two songs from backstage.

SAILING
Sutherland (Taken from the
album 459151: ATLANTIC CROSSING)

A

RPM
6800

Island
Music Ltd
Manufactured
in the UK

ROD STEWART
Produced by Tom Dowd

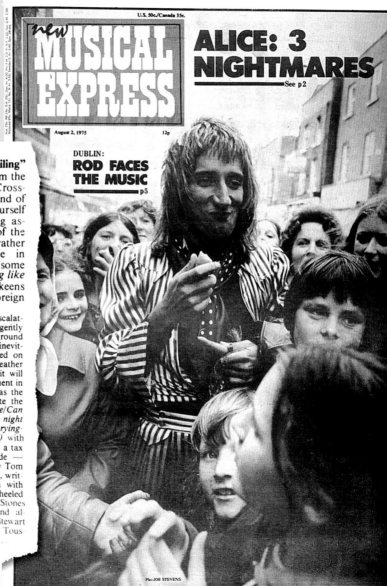

new MUSICAL EXPRESS

U.S. 50c/Canada 35c.

August 2, 1975   12p

ALICE: 3 NIGHTMARES

See p 2

DUBLIN:
ROD FACES THE MUSIC

p 5

ROD STEWART: "Sailing" (Warner Bros.). Lifted from the forthcoming "Atlantic Crossing" lp, "Sailing" is the kind of tune you might find yourself having to sing in morning assembly. Written by one of the Sutherland Bros., it's a rather dreary sentimental piece in which Mr. Stewart, via some very basic imagery (*"flying like a bird 'cross the sky"*), keens for his loved one in foreign parts.

The chord progressions and escalating heavenly chorale swaying gently with scarves aloft in the background suggest that at any moment the inevitable rent-a-piper will be wheeled on brandishing bouquets of heather wrapped in tin foil. Doubtless it will prove to be a Very Moving Moment in some forthcoming stage show as the audience will naturally associate the lyrics (sample: *"Can you hear me/Can you hear me/Through the dark night far away/I am dying/Forever crying To be with you/Who can say?"*) with Stewart's homesickness at being a tax exile in Hollywood. The B side — again rather poorly produced by Tom Dowd — is "Stone Cold Sober", written by Stewart in conjunction with Steve Cropper, and is a drag-heeled garage band re-run in the Stones "Happy" tradition. Might sound alright if you're drunk. Maybe Stewart should have worked with Allen Toussaint after all. Talking of whom . . .

Pic: JOE STEVENS

100

Mississippi
Pussycat

Release Date: 28.08.76
No. Weeks In Chart: 22
Reached No. 1: 16.10.76
Total Sales: 947,000

'Mississippi' was Pussycat's only No. 1 record, the pinnacle of a fleeting two-hit career.

Hailing from Limburg, in Holland, Pussycat were the first Dutch act to make it to the UK top spot.

The group was made up of two daughters of a Polish miner – the girls were previously known as The Singing Sisters – along with Toni and Lou Wille, who were still working day jobs just prior to the single's chart-topping success.

Four male musicians were brought in from a hard-rock act called Scum, and a deal with EMI was signed, which produced this surprise smash single, a chart-topper in Europe, New Zealand and Africa as well as the UK.

Despite the lack of Top 20 hits after their follow-up single, 'Smile', had reached No. 24 in December of that year, the group stayed together for a number of years and released another six albums, which sold solidly in their homeland and other parts of Europe.

'Mississippi' sold more than seven million copies globally, and even managed to stay on one South American chart for two and a half years.

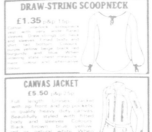

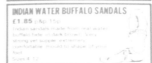

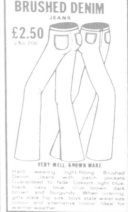

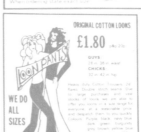

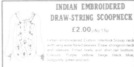

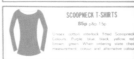

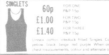

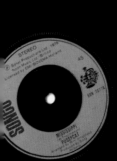

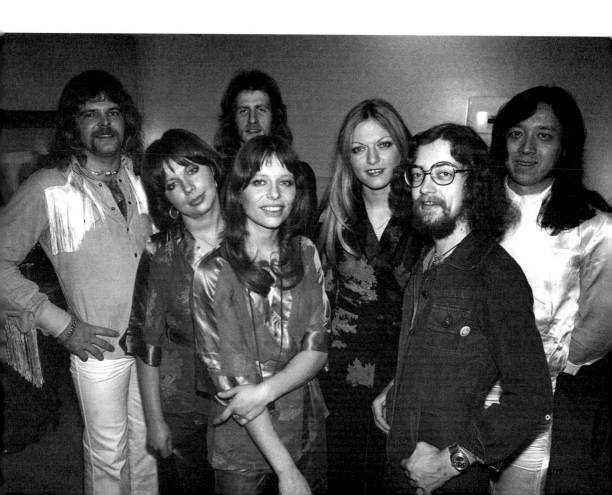

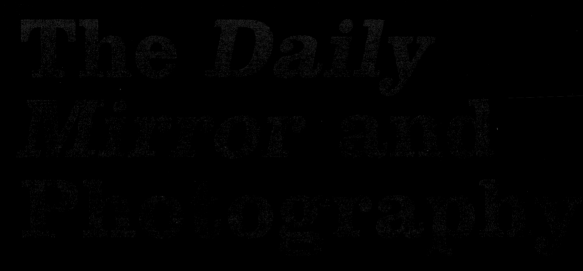

The *Daily Mirror* and Photography

Music and the media have been inextricably linked since the very beginnings of rock 'n' roll.

Up until the '50s, politicians and current affairs had hogged the front pages of national newspapers, their reign interrupted only by the occasional special feature on film stars, the latter being by far the highest profile entertainers of the day.

However, when records by performers such as Elvis, Bill Haley and Jerry Lee Lewis started arriving on these shores, newspapers immediately picked up on the sales potential of the burgeoning teenage market, to whom – until now – the press had done little to appeal.

Throughout the '50s, popular culture was dominated by American imports; but by the dawn of the '60s, Britain was ready to fight

back. There was a palpable sense of expectation as Fleet Street poised itself to champion new British acts. One act over and above all others spearheaded this early explosion of British music, and the media adored them: they were, of course, The Beatles.

In Fleet Street, the *Daily Mirror* was perfectly placed to capture the genuine cultural phenomenon that was Beatlemania. In those days, the newspaper employed over twenty staff photographers, way in excess of the streamlined freelance networks of today. Each and every one of the *Mirror*'s staffers photographed The Beatles, most of them taking three sessions or more, thereby bequeathing to

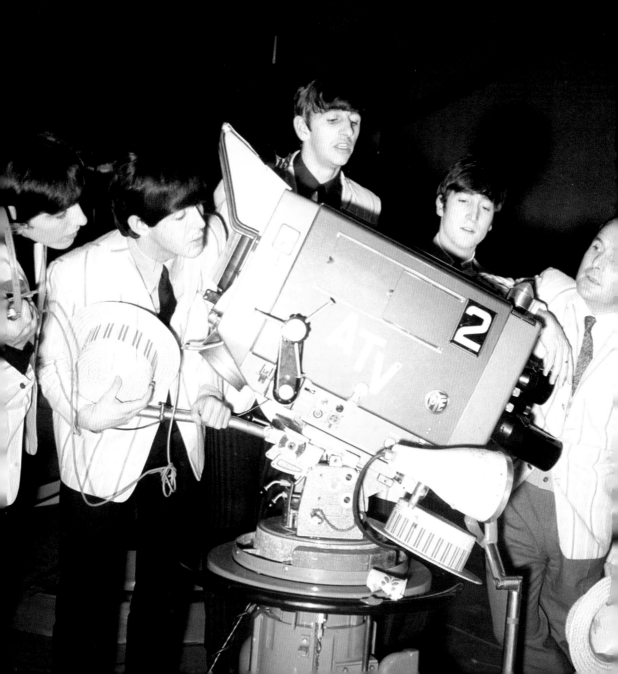

this newspaper a unique archive of both reportage and posed Beatles' pictures.

Victor Crawshaw and Alisdair MacDonald took many of the most famous shots, often at airports, sometimes live or on tour overseas. MacDonald even captured one of John and Yoko's 'bed-ins' at the Amsterdam Hilton. The *Mirror* staff photographers were nothing if not adaptable; they might one night be capturing the Fab Four surrounded by thousands of screaming fans; but the next day, if a news story required, for example, a trip to the East End to snap a murder scene or a local jamboree, they would cover that, too.

The challenges of photographing The Beatles at that early stage are in sharp contrast to those faced by the celebrity photographers of today. Invariably, the lighting was of poor quality; the photographers' high-quality lenses were not assisted by electronic or digital capabilities, while venues and even band managers were not always as accommodating as one might expect. Interestingly, MacDonald recalls in the book *The Beatles Files* (CLB

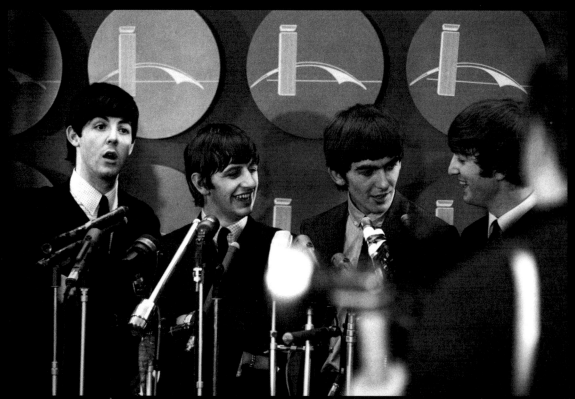

...international, 1998) now they were more intent on photographing from behind the band than from in front. 'Nobody was very interested in the Beatles at first! The stories weren't so much about them, but what happens around them. We'd mainly stand with our backs to the stage photographing the kids. All the paper wanted to see were these hysterical swooning girls.' Back in those days, bands were also not averse to posing with a copy of the *Daily Mirror* in their hands.

Fast forward to Reading Festival 2002. The Foo Fighters, featuring ex-Nirvana drummer Dave Grohl, are headlining the Saturday night bill. The 50,000-strong crowd in the field in Berkshire is going ballistic. Unknown to the screaming fans, right down at the front of the stage in a muddied section of grass – between the band and the thick-set security guards holding back the crowd – a far more frantic mêlée is taking place, making the fabled 'mosh pit' seem rather tame. A gaggle of photographers are fighting to get their pictures, using aluminium stepladders, beer crates, even each other to clamber into position.

After three songs, the photographers are escorted away – standard practice for a band of The Foo Fighters' size. Backstage, band members of such huge groups are usually hurried through to their dressing room. However, splintering off from the tunnel of escorts, Dave Grohl greets fans and lets them take snaps. There are no newspaper photographers backstage.

These days, a *Mirror* photographer might ...

closer to the most elusive celebrities. Each snap is taken digitally and then beamed across the Internet at lightning speed for use within seconds. Back in 1963 when the *Daily Mirror* men were snapping The Beatles, film and prints would have to be couriered back to HQ or, if the photographers were overseas, sent by freight.

The focus of the *Mirror* pictures has changed too. Live shots are used much more rarely. The newspaper's celebrity page, *3am*, focuses on celebrity lifestyle and uses an extensive network of contacts to bring in exclusive stories on high-profile names in music, film and entertainment.

The brief for the *Daily Mirror* is also much wider in these modern times, taking in worldwide acts, global superstars, parties in New York and London in the same paragraph and using snaps of stars from all over the world on the same page. Yet the secret of success remains the same – the instinctive reaction of the photographer to seize a specific moment in time, a millisecond of history before it is lost forever. That skill will always outweigh any amount of technology and equipment.

However, although big-name acts enjoy spells of dominating the entertainment pages, no other act since The Beatles has enjoyed such an intimate relationship with a newspaper. As Alisdair MacDonald summarised, 'You could go out and do a baby picture or an animal picture but when you got back to the office they'd say they already had one . . . but The Beatles pictures went straight in. With them we couldn't fail. They sold newspapers and the ...

Chart Facts and Stats

Male Artists With The Most No. 1s

1 . Elvis Presley (18)   ● ● ● ● ● ● ● ● ● ● ● ● ● ● ● ● ● ●

2 . Cliff Richard (14)   ● ● ● ● ● ● ● ● ● ● ● ● ● ●

3 . = Michael Jackson (7)   ● ● ● ● ● ● ●

3 . = George Michael (7)   ● ● ● ● ● ● ●

4 . Rod Stewart (6)   ● ● ● ● ● ●

Female Artists With The Most No. 1s

1 . Madonna (10)   ● ● ● ● ● ● ● ● ● ●

2 . Kylie Minogue (6)   ● ● ● ● ● ●

3 . = Whitney Houston (4)   ● ● ● ●

3 . = Geri Halliwell (4)   ● ● ● ●

4 . = Billie Piper (3)   ● ● ●

4 . = Britney Spears (3)   ● ● ●

4 . = Sandie Shaw (3)   ● ● ●

4 . = Cher (3)   ● ● ●

4 . = Olivia Newton-John (3)   ● ● ●

Chart Facts and Stats

Most Consecutive Weeks At No. 1

1. Bryan Adams – (Everything I Do) I Do It For You (16 weeks) – (1991)

2. Wet Wet Wet – Love Is All Around (15 weeks) – (1994)

3. Slim Whitman – Rose Marie (11 weeks) – (1955)

4. = Whitney Houston – I Will Always Love You (10 weeks) – (1992)

4. = David Whitfield – Cara Mia (10 weeks) – (1954)

Bands With The Most No. 1s

1. The Beatles (17) ● ● ● ● ● ● ● ● ● ● ● ● ● ● ● ● ●

2. Westlife (10) ● ● ● ● ● ● ● ● ● ●

3. Abba (9) ● ● ● ● ● ● ● ● ●

4. Spice Girls (9) ● ● ● ● ● ● ● ● ●

5. = Rolling Stones (8) ● ● ● ● ● ● ● ●

5. = Take That (8) ● ● ● ● ● ● ● ●

Million-Selling Singles

The following singles have all sold more than one million copies in the UK.

Note: Dates refer to the year in which the track sold its millionth copy.
This can differ significantly from the year of release/peak chart success.

Year	Title	Artist
1957	Rock Around The Clock	Bill Haley & His Comets
1957	Diana	Paul Anka
1957	Mary's Boy Child	Harry Belafonte
1960	It's Now Or Never	Elvis Presley
1962	Stranger On The Shore	Mr Acker Bilk
1962	I Remember You	Frank Ifield
1962	The Young Ones	Cliff Richard & The Shadows
1963	She Loves You	The Beatles
1963	I Want To Hold Your Hand	The Beatles
1964	Can't Buy Me Love	The Beatles
1964	I Feel Fine	The Beatles
1965	The Carnival Is Over	The Seekers
1965	Tears	Ken Dodd
1965	We Can Work It Out/Day Tripper	The Beatles
1966	Green, Green Grass Of Home	Tom Jones
1967	Release Me	Englebert Humperdinck
1967	The Last Waltz	Englebert Humperdinck
1974	I Love You Love Me Love	Gary Glitter
1975	Bohemian Rhapsody	Queen
1976	Save Your Kisses For Me	Brotherhood of Man
1976	Don't Give Up On Us	David Soul
1977	White Christmas	Bing Crosby
1978	Mull Of Kintyre/Girls' School	Paul McCartney & Wings
1978	Eye Level	The Simon Park Orchestra
1978	Rivers Of Babylon/ Brown Girl In The Ring	Boney M
1978	Mary's Boy Child - Oh My Lord	Boney M
1978	You're The One That I Want	John Travolta & Olivia Newton-John
1979	YMCA	Village People
1979	Heart Of Glass	Blondie
1979	Bright Eyes	Art Garfunkel
1979	Summer Nights	John Travolta and Olivia Newton-John
1980	Merry Xmas Everybody	Slade
1981	Imagine	John Lennon
1981	Tainted Love	Soft Cell
1982	Don't You Want Me	Human League
1982	Come On Eileen	Dexy's Midnight Runners

Year	Title	Artist
1983	Karma Chameleon	Culture Club
1983	Blue Monday	New Order
1984	Relax	Frankie Goes To Hollywood
1984	Careless Whisper	George Michael
1984	Two Tribes	Frankie Goes To Hollywood
1984	I Just Called To Say I Love You	Stevie Wonder
1984	Do They Know It's Christmas	Band Aid
1985	Last Christmas / Everything She Wants	Wham!
1985	The Power Of Love	Jennifer Rush
1991	(Everything I Do) I Do It For You	Bryan Adams
1993	I Will Always Love You	Whitney Houston
1994	Love Is All around	Wet Wet Wet
1994	Saturday Night	Whigfield
1994	Think Twice	Celine Dion
1995	Gangsta's Paradise	Coolio featuring LV
1995	Unchained Melody/ The White Cliffs Of Dover	Robson & Jerome
1995	I Believe/Up On The Roof	Robson & Jerome
1996	Earth Song	Michael Jackson
1996	Spaceman	Babylon Zoo
1996	Wannabe	Spice Girls
1996	Killing Me Softly	Fugees
1997	2 Become 1	Spice Girls
1997	I'll Be Missing You	Puff Daddy & Faith Evans
1997	Candle In The Wind '97	Elton John
1997	Barbie Girl	Aqua
1997	Perfect Day	Various Artists
1998	Teletubbies Say Eh-Oh	Teletubbies
1998	Never Ever	All Saints
1998	It's Like That	Jason Nevins vs Run-D.M.C.
1998	My Heart Will Go On	Celine Dion
1998	No Matter What	Boyzone
1998	Believe	Cher
1999	Heartbeat / Tragedy	Steps
1999	Baby One More Time	Britney Spears
1999	Blue (Da Ba Dee)	Eiffel 65
2001	Can We Fix It?	Bob the Builder
2001	Pure & Simple	Hear'Say
2001	It Wasn't Me	Shaggy featuring Rikrok
2002	Can't Get You Out Of My Head	Kylie Minogue
2002	Anything Is Possible/Evergreen	Will Young
2002	Unchained Melody	Gareth Gates

Christmas No. 1s

Artist	Song Title	Chart Week Ending Date	Weeks at No. 1
Al Martino	Here In My Heart	14/11/52	9
Frankie Laine	Answer Me	13/11/53	8
Winifred Atwell	Let's Have Another Party	3/12/54	5
Dickie Valentine	Christmas Alphabet	16/12/55	3
Johnnie Ray	Just Walking In The Rain	16/11/56	7
Harry Belafonte	Mary's Boy Child	22/11/57	7
Conway Twitty	It's Only Make Believe	19/12/58	5
Emile Ford & The Checkmates	What Do You Want To Make Those Eyes At Me For	18/12/59	6
Cliff Richard & The Shadows	I Love You	29/12/60	2
Danny Williams	Moon River	28/12/61	2
Elvis Presley	Return To Sender	13/12/62	3
Beatles	I Want To Hold Your Hand	12/12/63	5
Beatles	I Feel Fine	10/12/64	5
Beatles	Day Tripper/We Can Work It Out	16/12/65	5
Tom Jones	Green, Green Grass Of Home	1/12/66	7
Beatles	Hello, Goodbye	6/12/67	7
Scaffold	Lily The Pink	11/12/68 & 8/1/69	3 & 1
Rolf Harris	Two Little Boys	20/12/69	6
Dave Edmunds	I Hear You Knockin'	28/11/70	6
Benny Hill	Ernie (The Fastest Milkman In The West)	11/12/71	4
Little Jimmy Osmond	Long Haired Lover From Liverpool	23/12/72	5
Slade	Merry Xmas Everybody	15/12/73	5
Mud	Lonely This Christmas	21/12/74	4
Queen	Bohemian Rhapsody	29/11/75	9
Johnny Mathis	When A Child Is Born (Soleado)	25/12/76	3

Artist	Song Title	Chart Week Ending Date	Weeks at No. 1
Wings	Mull Of Kintyre/Girls' School	3/12/77	9
Boney M	Mary's Boy Child – Oh My Lord	9/12/78	4
Pink Floyd	Another Brick In The Wall (Part 2)	15/12/79	5
St Winifred's School Choir	There's No One Quite Like Grandma	27/12/80	2
Human League	Don't You Want Me	12/12/81	5
Renee & Renato	Save Your Love	18/12/82	4
Flying Pickets	Only You	10/12/83	5
Band Aid	Do They Know It's Christmas	15/12/84	5
Shakin' Stevens	Merry Christmas Everyone	28/12/85	2
Jackie Wilson	Reet Petite	27/12/86	4
Pet Shop Boys	Always On My Mind	19/12/87	4
Cliff Richard	Mistletoe & Wine	10/12/88	4
Band Aid II	Do They Know It's Christmas	23/12/89	3
Cliff Richard	Saviour's Day	22/12/90	1
Queen	Bohemian Rhapsody/ These Are The Days Of Our Lives	21/12/91	5
Whitney Houston	I Will Always Love You	5/12/92	10
Mr Blobby	Mr Blobby	11/12/93 & 25/12/93	1 & 2
East 17	Stay Another Day	10/12/94	5
Michael Jackson	Earth Song	9/12/95	6
Spice Girls	2 Become 1	28/12/96	3
Spice Girls	Too Much	27/12/97	2
Spice Girls	Goodbye	26/12/98	1
Westlife	I Have A Dream/ Seasons In The Sun	25/12/99	4
Bob The Builder	Can We Fix It	23/12/00	3
Robbie Williams and Nicole Kidman	Somethin' Stupid	22/12/01	3

Chart Facts and Stats

Bands With The Most Weeks In The Top 75

1. The Beatles – 456 weeks

2. Queen – 419 weeks

3. Status Quo – 413 weeks

4. The Rolling Stones – 366 weeks

5. The Shadows – 359 weeks*

*Excludes The Shadows with Cliff Richard.

Singles In This List Which Failed To Make No. 1

Wham!	Last Christmas/Everything She Wants – reached No. 2
Mr Acker Bilk	Stranger On The Shore – reached No. 2
New Order	Blue Monday – reached No. 3
Natalie Imbruglia	Torn – reached No. 2
Ray Parker Jr	Ghostbusters – reached No. 2
Oasis	Wonderwall – reached No. 2

About the List's Compilers:

Alan Jones

Alan Jones is one of the most respected commentators on the Official UK Charts. During a career that has spanned over twenty years, Alan has amassed an enormous archive of chart-related data, much of which has been used in the creation of this list of Top 100 Best-Selling Singles. In addition to being *Music Week*'s senior charts writer, he is the co-author of a number of specialist music publications.

Tony Brown

Tony Brown was editorial associate for the *Guinness Book of British Hit Singles* for ten years, from 1987 to 1997; from 1990 he also worked in the chart department of *Music Week*. Paul Gambaccini has described Tony as a 'chartologist par excellence'. Included among Tony's chart and music-related books are *The Complete Book of the British Charts* and *The Complete Eurovision Song Contest Companion*.

Acknowledgments

The author and publisher would like to thank Andy Linehan at the National Sound Archive of the British Library, for permission to photograph all of the vinyl singles appearing in this book.

Thanks are also due to all the staff at *NME* who provided assistance in researching the *NME* material for this book; and to the *NME* for allowing access to their archive.

Thanks also to Rob Dimery for stepping into the breach and providing invaluable editorial support.

Singles photography: Neil Sutherland
NME archive photography: Michael Wicks

Last, but not least, the author wishes to extend his heartfelt thanks to his wife, Kaye Roach, along with Deb Rumble and Simon Park.